Helping to Care

A handbook for carers at home
and in hospital

Helping to Care
A handbook for Carers at home and in hospital

by

Betty Kershaw
RGN, OND, DANS, RCNT, RNT, MSc (Nursing), CMS
Director of Nurse Education,
Stockport Health Authority.

Stephen G. Wright
RGN, RCNT, DipN, DANS, RNT, MSc (Nursing)
Consultant Nurse,
Nursing Development Unit,
Tameside General Hospital,
Ashton-under-Lyne.

and

Pauline Hammonds
RGN, SCM, NDN cert
Lecturer in Health Promotion and Health Studies,
Central Manchester College,
Openshaw Centre, Manchester.

Baillière Tindall
London Philadelphia Toronto Sydney Tokyo

Baillière Tindall
W. B. Saunders

24–28 Oval Road
London NW1 7DX, England

The Curtis Center
Independence Square West
Philadelphia, PA 19106–3399, USA

1 Goldthorne Avenue
Toronto, Ontario M8Z 5T9, Canada

Harcourt Brace Jovanovich Group (Australia) Pty Ltd
32–52 Smidmore Street
Marrickville, NSW 2204, Australia

Harcourt Brace Jovanovich Japan Inc.
Ichibancho Central Building, 22–1 Ichibancho
Chiyoda-ku, Tokyo 102, Japan

First published 1989

British Library Cataloguing in Publication Data

Kershaw, Betty
  Helping to care.
  1. Great Britain. Hospitals. Long stay
  patients. Care   2. Great Britain. Dependent
  persons. Home care
  I. Title   II. Wright, Steve   III. Hammonds,
  Pauline
  362.1'1'0941

  ISBN 0-7020-1337-4

Typeset by Colset Private Limited, Singapore
Printed in Great Britain by Mackays of Chatham Plc, Chatham, Kent.

Contents

Contents

Introduction

As we move towards the 1990's more and more people are providing care for relatives and neighbours within their own homes. Others are giving voluntary support in hospitals and community homes and an increasing number are finding paid employment in health care or social work settings. Having to accept one's role as a carer can be traumatic if you have never done it before. People are often unaware of how to seek help, and which professionals are available to assist them. This small but comprehensive book aims to address the problems faced by carers, and to enable carers to assist patients, family members, neighbours or friends to adapt to the changes age, ill-health or handicap bring, with the goal of helping them achieve the best possible quality of life.

Increasingly, hospitals, and colleges of further education, are offering short courses to help carers develop caring skills, and, within the next two or three years those seeking paid employment as carers will be able to train for these jobs (currently called Support Worker posts) through specially prepared and validated vocational qualifications. As yet those courses are still at planning stages, but hospitals and colleges will have further information available by summer 1989. This book is no alternative to undertaking such a course; however, it does seek to provide a framework for safe practice and hopefully will be accepted by carers as a source of readily available information and advice, particularly when the trained nurse or social worker is not at hand.

1

The management of care

Whether you work as a nursing auxiliary in hospital or in patients' homes, your day to day work is supervised by qualified nurses. If you work in an Aged Persons' Home you are part of the caring team employed by the social services. If you are one of the many people who care for relatives and friends, or give your time as a volunteer, you will be only too aware of the many different care workers you meet.

The aim of this introductory chapter is to explain who else is involved in giving care, how the delivery of care is managed, and how you fit into the caring team.

Ninety per cent of persons receiving care and treatment through the National Health Service (NHS) in this country today (1988) are being cared for at home. The figure is even higher for those people who receive support from the social services. It is therefore most appropriate to look first at the structure of care in the community.

The community nursing team

District nurse

The district nurse is a registered nurse who has undertaken further studies for the National District Nursing (NDN) certificate, which prepares her* to work in people's homes. She is an

---

*The predominant use of 'she' when referring to care workers and 'he' when referring to the patient is merely for convenience and does not deny the existence of male nurses or female patients!

extremely skilled nursing practitioner and is capable of working alone, making decisions, directing a team and assisting patients and relatives to live in their own homes where possible. In some health authorities she is based in health centres; in others she works from her own home. In both cases she works closely with the patient's general practitioner (GP) and is responsible to a senior nurse. Her team will probably include an enrolled nurse and a nursing auxiliary but may consist of registered nurses not yet holding the NDN certificate but waiting for a course place.

The district nurse will carry the case load and will see all her patients at regular intervals. Those in need of expert care she will care for herself, for example those who need frequent injections of dangerous drugs. Otherwise she will delegate care to her enrolled nurse and either directly or indirectly to the auxiliary.

Community enrolled nurse

Like all enrolled nurses, community enrolled nurses are directed by a registered nurse but are trusted and relied upon to give care as directed and to seek guidance from the registered nurse when needed.

Auxiliary nurse/bath attendant

Some community teams employ unqualified staff to assist in those aspects of care often provided by relatives or friends. These include bathing, dressing, undressing and ensuring that those who live alone are comfortable for the night. The district nurse, whether enrolled or registered, will direct and monitor care, visiting the patient and the auxiliary nurse regularly to ensure that she carries out her duties as directed and that she reports any change in the patient's condition or anything else that she feels is important. Training is often given so that the assistant becomes capable and competent in giving necessary care.

The hospital nursing team

Ward sister or charge nurse

Like the district nurse, the ward sister (or charge nurse if male) is a registered nurse. She may have undertaken a further nursing course in her special area of nursing interest and she will have considerable experience in nursing patients with the specific conditions found on her ward. She works closely with the consultants and their medical teams and directs the work of her nursing staff.

Staff nurse

Staff nurses have studied for three years for the Registered General Nurse (RGN) qualification. They run the ward in the sister's absence and are responsible for the care of patients in the ward.

Enrolled nurse

Enrolled nurses follow a two-year programme. They are prepared by their training to give care under the supervision of the registered nurse and to assist her in the performance of more complicated nursing duties.

Auxiliary nurse

Auxiliary nurses are employed to assist the nursing staff and to help patients with basic activities of living, such as washing, eating and going to the toilet, and to do other tasks as directed by the nursing staff. Many hospitals have training programmes for their auxiliary nurses and it is advisable to join one of these courses if possible.

Staff who work in both hospital and community

The ward sister and district nurse co-ordinate medical treatment and treatment that the patient receives from para-medical staff, such as occupational therapists or physiotherapists. All services provided in hospital, including dentistry and speech therapy, are available for patients in the community.

Senior nurse

Senior nurses are appointed from experienced ward sisters or district nurses (or, where appropriate, from midwives or psychiatric nurses) to provide expert clinical advice and to manage, for example, a group of several wards or a community health centre.

Physiotherapist

The physiotherapist has completed a three-year degree or diploma course. Her special skills are in maintaining physiological functions and ensuring that the patient is ambulant to the best of his or her ability, or helping those who have difficulty breathing to breathe more easily by using all their muscles. Physiotherapists are especially valuable when patients need active rehabilitation and they also teach relatives and friends to help.

Occupational therapist

The occupational therapist has followed either a four-year degree programme, or a three-year diploma course. She works with patients and their families to develop new skills, such as using special cooking items following a stroke, or using dressing aids for those who are physically impaired. Occupational therapists also encourage patients to enjoy recreational activities, such as music and painting, which encourage relaxation and the development of new interests.

Chiropodists

Chiropodists are professionals who provide treatment for foot problems. They are frequently consulted when patients have difficulty walking, because of corns and bunions, for example, and are often required to treat ingrowing toenails. Diabetic patients are especially prone to foot infections; a chiropodist should always be consulted when these patients have foot problems.

Liaison nurse

The liaison nurse is the key person in co-ordinating care between the hospital and community. She is an expert hospital and community nurse and is responsible for arranging a patient's discharge from hospital, to ensure a smooth transition of care. She will arrange transport and clinic appointments, for example, and check that necessary drugs and appliances are available.

Health visitor

The health visitor may be part of the community or the child health unit. Most of her work is concerned with children under five, but increasingly she is becoming involved in providing health advice for the elderly who need her help to maintain health. The health visitor is an RGN with midwifery experience and a year's further study.

Community psychiatric nurse

The community psychiatric nurse's role is also discussed in Chapter 16. Although usually employed with the psychiatric unit, she works closely with the community nursing team.

Caring for patients in the community is made easier by day centres or by short-term admission to hospital. Both offer a respite to full-time carers and enable the patient to benefit from special services more readily available in hospital. Rehabilitation can be encouraged and such services as chiropody and hairdressing are often available. A small charge may be made if these services are not ordered by a physician. Patients with special problems may also receive advice, for example on dental care.

The nursing process

Many ward sisters and district nurses use the nursing process for planning and delivering patient care. The nursing process is a systematic approach which requires the nurse to identify the problems that the patient (and family) are experiencing due to their state of health, and to plan necessary care to resolve the problem. The nurse must discuss care and treatment with the patient, family and friends, as well as with other members of the health care team. The health care team is made up of those health care professionals who are involved with a particular patient; thus each patient's care team may differ. Each team includes a doctor and nurse but not all will include paramedics.

The nurse knows which members of the health care team to consult and adds their information to that obtained from conversations with the patient and next of kin. This enables her to identify the problems the patient is experiencing and therefore to plan and implement appropriate nursing action to ensure that the patient's needs are met.

Let us consider how the nursing process works in action by looking at a patient who has just been admitted to a geriatric rehabilitation unit.

Mr Simon Jones is 82 and lives alone in a ground floor council flat. His son lives close by and calls every day but is unwilling to shop or provide any physical care. Four weeks ago Mr Jones fell and broke his left wrist. Although the fracture has healed, mobility of the joint is not fully restored and he has daily physiotherapy. He has been admitted, at the request of his GP, for active rehabilitation to give him confidence in caring for himself. Since his fall he has become frightened of moving and falling and sits in a chair all day. He has had the occasional incontinent accident during the day, although at night he has no problems, since he keeps a bottle by his bed. He has no problems with writing or eating since he is right-handed.

The assessing nurse identifies his nursing needs:

- To gain confidence in his ability to walk and to care for himself.
- To increase mobility and strength in his wrist.
- To resolve his incontinence (which she decides is related to his mobility problem).

A care plan is prepared which enables him to build up confidence. Each day the nurse encourages him to walk a little further and to use a stick—prepared for him by the physiotherapy department—to help him with support. Initially the physiotherapist teaches him how to use the stick and the nurses reinforce this in day to day movement around the ward.

He is receiving daily physiotherapy for his wrist. On the suggestion of the sister, the nurse mentions the problem to the occupational therapist who supports her. He is encouraged to play cards and other games using that hand. This helps, especially when the nurse responsible for his care remembers to remind him to do his exercises.

His incontinence problem also improves as he gains confidence in his mobility. After two weeks the care given is evaluated and found to be successful. It is relatively easy now to return Mr Jones to his home but the staff want to ensure that once home he receives some support.

The community liaison nurse visits and suggests that a visit to a local authority day centre might be possible once a week. She also knows of a voluntary society lunch club near to his flat. She, in turn, contacts the social services who can arrange one day a week at the day centre. They can also co-ordinate transport through volunteer services. Once he is home they agree to see if there are other services that can be provided to help him.

When you consider the action the nurse must take it becomes clear that those members of the nursing care teams cannot meet all the patient's needs. It is therefore necessary to involve the social services.

The social services

A care assistant working for the social services could work in an Aged Persons' Home, in a hostel for the mentally or physically handicapped, in a children's home, as a home help, or with one of the voluntary organisations. For example social service departments often allocate the money for 'Meals on Wheels' to the WRVS (Women's Royal Voluntary Services) who may employ staff to help.

In any of these posts the care assistant will be responsible to a qualified social worker, often a graduate with specialist qualifications in the field in which she supervises. If someone is caring for a friend or relative at home, the social worker will visit should the need arise. Social workers also work in hospitals, where they often have responsibility for a special area of care, for example child or maternity patients. Social workers are responsible to directors who have considerable practical and management experience and advanced training.

The UK is divided into social service authorities which cover the same areas as counties. At local level there is a local authority social service department linked with local authority boundaries. These are not always the same as health authority boundaries, so that a member of a community nursing team may be seeing patients who receive support from different social service departments. Similarly a social worker in a hospital may be referring patients to different departments too.

Social workers are the best people to advise patients and families about benefits available through the social security system. If the care assistant suspects that a patient has financial worries, or that extra money may be needed because of illness or treatment, the immediate superior should be told so that the social worker can be asked to visit. Help with pensions and grants may also be obtainable from charitable associations. Like all other information concerning patients, their financial support must remain confidential.

The management of the services which fund and deliver health care is complicated. Figure 1.1 explains how the social services are administered at local level. The social services are responsible to the Department of Health (DH) and the Department of Social Security (DSS). The NHS is also responsible to the DH and DSS; both receive their funding from taxation. Figure 1.2 illustrates the structure of the NHS within a district health authority (DHA).

The national health service

The NHS is responsible for all services relating to the care of the sick or the maintenance of health. This includes providing (a) necessary hospital out-patient clinics and staff (doctors, nurses, midwives, physiotherapists, auxiliary nurses, etc) to care for those who are ill and (b) adequate welfare clinics, diagnostic services, GPs and school nurses—to name but a few—to promote and maintain good health. Family planning and maternity services are also provided by the NHS. There are, of course, services other than the NHS who accept responsibility for caring

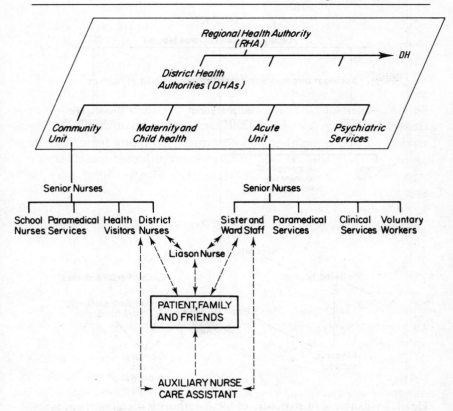

Fig. 1.1 Example of structure within a district health authority. Health visitors may be placed in the community or child health unit, since their role covers aspects of both. Similarly, nurses caring for the mentally handicapped may be in either psychiatric or community units.

for the sick and maintaining health. These include the armed services, who run their own hospitals, and many industrial and business concerns, who provide an occupational health service for their staff. There are also the private health care organisations, who do not obtain their funds from the NHS budget but from fees and subscriptions. Auxiliary nurses may, therefore, be employed outside the NHS.

For most people in this country, however, health care is provided through the NHS on a regional basis. There are 14 regional health authorities (RHAs) in England which vary in area since

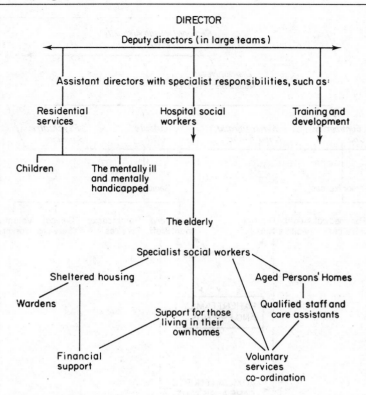

Fig. 1.2 Example of structure of local authority social services team.

they are based on population density. Thus the regions that have large populations, such as the London regions and the north-western region, which serves Manchester and Preston, are much smaller in area than the RHAs that cover less populated counties. The south-western region stretches from Land's End to the villages north and east of Bristol. Regional spread based on population is one way of allocating services 'fairly' but it does mean that those services provided on a regional basis (such as open heart surgery and paediatric cancer care) are much further from home than if you live in one of the more densely populated regions. The NHS recognises this, and although a patient is normally expected to attend for treatment within his or her home region, arrangements can be made for patients to cross regional boundaries when this is more convenient for them and their families.

A restructuring of the management of services at local level was completed by late 1987 and all RHAs now have a regional general manager, who accepts responsibility for the management of the NHS facilities within his or her region. These regional general managers receive advice from specialist professionals including a senior nurse. Similarly each DHA has a district general manager, who divides the district into units (for example a community unit, an acute services unit), each with a unit general manager. These district and unit managers may be nurses; if not, legislation requires the general manager to appoint a nurse to advise on nursing matters.

The appropriate unit general manager is responsible for appointing ward sisters, health visitors and district nurses who work with patients and their families. They, in turn, are often responsible for appointing those who will work with them, including auxiliary nurses, and it is these registered nurses who will direct and monitor the work of more junior staff. Where appropriate they will also advise those who care for patients in their own homes.

Ward sisters and district nurses accept responsibility for ensuring that those who work under their guidance deliver the best possible patient care. They do this by supervising and monitoring care given. Equally, they accept responsibility for ensuring that patients and, where appropriate, their families and friends are involved in decisions that relate to care and treatment. Patients and their families should also be taught how to give care themselves, for example an injection for a diabetic patient, or a bath or a shower for someone who is physically disabled.

Because of the many people and diverse services involved in ensuring that patients and families receive the best possible treatment and care, everyone must work closely together and respect the valuable job each is doing. Otherwise some aspect of care will be missed or forgotten, or there will be a duplication of services. Confidential communication is the key to cost-effective, efficient care. Write down what you do and ask advice if in doubt. In that way, everyone will be informed and all patients will receive the best available care—no more, no less.

2

The delivery of care

In recent years nurses have been looking much more closely at the philosophy of what they do. This may sound rather grand, but it is important to examine nurses self-perception, who they see as patients and how they work with them. Other professions have been doing the same sort of thing; we need to look at our underlying beliefs to see how they affect our day to day work as carers.

Broadly speaking, there could be said to be two types of approaches to care, at opposite ends of a spectrum, with varying shades in between. On the one hand, there is the approach that might be called 'mechanistic': patients are seen as objects and care is administered 'to' them. The patient's thoughts or feelings are taken into account very little. He or she is often seen as part of a large, homogeneous group, being treated in the same way according to the 'label' of his or her condition or disease. Sadly, this view has led to a very impersonal approach to care in many settings. It is often characterised by strict adherence (by patients and staff) to rules and regulations. Where such care is compounded by poor resources and staff education, then downright cruelty and ill treatment can ensue. This has often been exposed when major investigations have taken place (for example the Ely and Rampton enquiries). Martin (1984) identifies many such cases in his book (see 'Further Reading', p 176) and it might be a good idea to read this yourself. Unfortunately, it is feared that the official investigations only uncover the tip of the iceberg.

On the other end of the scale is the approach that we can call, for simplicity, 'humanistic'. Carers and patients or clients work much more as partners, with an understanding that the patient has rights. The patient's wishes and feelings are taken into account; he is treated much more as an individual with considerable freedom and choice in his care. The helper is encouraged to understand how the patient feels, to see things from the patient's point of view—in other words to *empathise* with the patient.

Our beliefs and values underpin very much the way we work with and approach the people we are caring for. The end results, at the extremes, are the two major patterns identified below. Where do you think you fit in with these? If you are doing your caring in a hospital, or some other institution, what pattern of care is being produced as a result of the staffs' efforts?

Try this simple exercise to help you think about it. Put a tick next to the following which applies to you/your setting:

Mechanistic/ institutionalised	*Humanistic/ individualised*
The hospital rules forbid parents to participate in their child's care. They are allowed to attend only at strict visiting times.	The parents are fully involved in the child's care, are taught to help by the nurses and can stay with him if they wish
A young disabled woman is fed, washed and has everything done for her by her carers. She tries to drink herself but is not allowed in case she spills.	She is given time to attempt to help herself and praised when she does. She is given the opportunity to do things for herself, like feeding, even at the risk of a mess or spillages.
An elderly man is admitted to hospital and has to bathe, eat and toilet at the times set by the nurses.	He is able to choose his own time for toiletting and bathing. The nurses ensure he has a choice of meals, and encourage relatives to provide foods he prefers at home which the hospital cannot supply.

The above exercise may help you think about your own approach to care. Perhaps there is a good rule in the old adage: 'Do unto others as you would have them do unto you'.

We all tend to prefer to be treated as individuals and to have our wishes taken into account when decisions are made about our health. The carer who empathises with a patient is better able to do this. While there are times when we might be happy to surrender our care into the hands of others (especially when we are very ill or helpless), this should not remove our right to have choice in that care, or the right to know how we are being helped and why. Think back to when you were last ill for any length of time and how it felt to be dependent. This book emphasises very much the individualised approach to care, because the authors themselves are very much affected by their own belief systems—beliefs as to who patients are and how best to help them. You will notice that there is a strong emphasis on carers *helping* or *assisting* with care rather than administering it to patients as if they are some sort of inanimate object.

The following definition of nursing offered by Virginia Henderson (1966) underpins the approach to care in this book:

'The unique function of the nurse is to assist the individual, sick or well, in the performance of those activities contributing to health or its recovery (or to a peaceful death) that he would perform unaided if he had the necessary strength, will or knowledge, and to do this in such a way as to help gain independence as rapidly as possible.'

Activities of living

So, we are in the business of *assisting* people to be as *independent* as they can be. To do this we are helping with those activities which people normally undertake themselves to be healthy, whilst appreciating how they feel about having to be helped. Henderson (1966) and Roper, Logan and Tierney (1986) identified groups of these activities; Wright (1986) has modified these activities in his work with the elderly (Table 2.1). You will notice that they help to form the structure of this book and later we will look at each activity in detail.

Table 2.1 The activities of living — a basis for problem solving

Creating and maintaining a safe environment
  comfort
  freedom from pain
  avoiding injury and infection
Communicating
  verbal and non-verbal
  forming interpersonal relationships
  expressing emotions, needs, fears, anxieties
  dealing with emotions of self and important others
  understanding how others feel (empathising)
  identifying/accepting positive and negative expressions, feelings,
    reactions
  maintaining and awareness of the environment
  using smell, touch, taste, hearing, seeing
Breathing
  meeting body oxygen needs
  maintaining a clear airway
  maintaining lung expansion
Eating and drinking
  maintaining nutritional requirements
  eating a balanced diet: vitamins, minerals, fats, carbohydrates,
    protein, roughage
  getting food to the mouth, chewing, swallowing, absorbing
  taking adequate fluids, maintaining hydration
  maintaining fluid/electrolyte balance
Eliminating
  passing urine and faeces
  maintaining normal and regular functioning
Personal cleansing and dressing
  skin, hair, nails
  mouth, teeth, eyes, ears
  selecting suitable clothing
  dressing/undressing
Maintaining normal body temperature
  sweating
  adjusting clothing
  environmental control
Working and playing
  having a sense of accomplishment
  enjoying recreation, hobbies, pastimes

Table 2.1 *Continued*

having a sense of worth and independence
participation in care and rehabilitation
Sexualising
  reproducing
  expressing sexuality, fulfilling needs
Resting and sleeping
  enjoying a normal sleep pattern
  taking desired rest periods
  promoting restful environment without stress, noise, anxiety
Learning
  discovering and satisfying curiosity
  developing normally
  acquiring knowledge and skills
  having a sense of achievement, facilitating awareness of self as an
    individual
  using knowledge and experience to maintain health and other
    activities
  learning to care for self — body and mind
  perceiving and acting on factors that influence health/illness
  making use of available health facilities
  accepting realistic goals in view of physical/mental limitations
Worshipping
  according to faith
  progressing towards personal spiritual goals
  using faith/beliefs as a source of reassurance in illness
Dying
  peacefully, without stress, pain or anxiety
  achieving final goals, accepting death
  needs met, needs of important others met

From Wright (1986) Building and Using a Model of Nursing (Edward Arnold, London).

Problem solving

When we are helping people we are spending much of our time problem solving. We work out what their difficulties are and decide what we hope to achieve and how we might achieve it with them; then we put our care into action and check that it is working satisfactorily.

- Assess (find out)
- Plan (decide what to do)
- Give care
- Evaluate (check that what we are doing is working)

As we evaluate our actions we may change our plan. Thus care can be a continuous activity or *'process'*. You may often hear the term 'nursing process', especially if you are working with nurses in the hospital or community. A full discussion on this subject is beyond the scope of this book (see 'Further reading', p 176, if you want to know more). Suffice to say this is a simple problem solving approach to care and is really the role of the trained nurse. Care plans can be passed on verbally and in writing to guide you in what you have to do. You, too, have a valuable contribution to make. What you learn about a patient can add much to the overall assessment and evaluation, and you may often be helping the trained nurse in the giving of care. Trained nurses bring an added depth of knowledge to the problem solving approach; in a strictly *nursing* setting you should always work under their guidance and seek their advice and assistance if in doubt.

Problem solving, however, is something we all do in our daily lives; as a carer you will often be involved in helping people with their health problems when they are less able to make decisions or carry out actions themselves. Remember, however, that your role is that of an *assistant* in care and you should not get yourself into a position where you are taking over the work that a trained professional should be carrying out or supervising. *When in doubt, ask!* You could ask those you work with—much will depend upon the kind of working relationships that are the norm in your setting. Alternatively, seek advice from relevant professionals (e.g. nurses, social workers, health visitors, the GP), trade union organisations and the many other organisations which offer advice relevant to your situation.

Organising care

In general, the way you go about giving care will be determined by the setting of the people you work with. There are many different patterns available. We tend to choose the methods which

- Get the job done
- Give the patients most satisfaction
- Give ourselves the most job satisfaction.

The ideal, of course, is to achieve all three goals. To this end nurses use different working methods, described below.

Task allocation

Sadly, some nurses still practise task allocation, in which each nurse is given a list of jobs to do, usually according to skill level and seniority. For example one nurse does the 'medicines', another the dressings and another tidies the beds. Hence care is often disjointed and confusing to both patient and nurse.

Team nursing

Small groups of nurses looking after small groups of patients. The team leader is usually a registered nurse. Often some elements of task allocation are involved, the more junior members doing the more menial tasks.

Patient allocation

One or two nurses are allocated to care for a limited number of patients, usually for a full shift of duty or perhaps longer.

Primary nursing

A nurse (registered) takes 24 hour responsibility for the care of a patient during his or her stay, in hospital and perhaps beyond.

None of the above working methods may apply to you if you are caring for someone at home on your own. You probably have a better chance then of making sure that the care you give your patient is very individualised and takes into account the patient's point of view. To a greater or lesser extent, all the above systems will require you to work as part of a team. Whatever method is used, you should bear in mind three rules:

- *Personalised* care should be given in any approach. If it is not, you will need to raise the issue (tactfully!) with your

colleagues to see how it might be organised differently. Some
systems (e.g. task allocation) are much more likely to leave the
patient feeling confused and uncertain, particularly when
many different nurses do different things to him. Again, you
will need to read some of the relevant texts if you want to discuss these methods in more detail.

- *Communication* within the team is vital. You must double
  check with your senior colleagues if you are unsure of what
  action to take. Reporting what you observe and what you do,
  or making your suggestions, are vital in ensuring the patient
  gets care of good quality and good continuity. Your contribution *is* valuable.

- *Confidentiality* must be maintained within the team. What
  you observe or what patients tell you must remain exclusive to
  you, your patient and your colleagues in the team. Pro-
  fessionally qualified colleagues must be kept informed of what
  patients tell you or of things you have observed relevant to
  their well-being. Your knowledge of patients, however,
  should not go beyond these boundaries. Talking about
  patients outside work to friends or acquaintances is not only
  extremely unethical, it may leave you open to serious charges
  of misconduct or even legal action. There is nothing wrong
  with talking in a general sense outside of work about what you
  do but you must be very careful not to cross that fine dividing
  line where you disclose private details of your patients or
  colleagues to outsiders.

  As a carer you will have access to many documents about
patients. These should only be used to help you organise your
care better, through an understanding of the patient and the
patient's needs. If you are employed as a carer, in hospital,
nursing home or community, you have a responsibility to use
such knowledge wisely to the benefit of your patients. In
general, you should only work under the direction of a trained
colleague. For the most part you are unlikely to encounter any
difficulties. However, you may occasionally find that a real
moral dilemma presents itself to you, especially when the rules
given above on communication and confidentiality come into
conflict.

  What do you do if a patient tells you something, in

confidence, which you fear may affect his health? What do you do if the patient tells you, again in confidence, of a serious criminal act that he has kept hidden? These and other problems like them may crop up to confront you as a carer from time to time, regardless of the setting in which you work. You may find it useful to raise such issues in discussion groups with colleagues to get a clearer picture in your mind of what action you must follow. If you have any doubts concerning serious dilemmas like this in your caring, you must discuss them with a senior (trained) professional. You may be able to discuss the issue in a general way without referring to your patient specifically or you may be able to seek advice from an outside professional or counsellor who is not involved.

Summary

We have taken a look at ways in which we must think about and organise our caring. Well thought out and well planned care is infinitely better than a jumbled and irrational chaos of actions—for both carers and cared for. It is true to say that how we do things is just as important as what we do.

3

Creating and maintaining a safe environment

We are all beset by hazards in our daily lives. Most of us are able to cope with the dangers from potential sources of injury and infection quite adequately. However, when someone is incapacitated—either mentally or physically—they may be unaware of or unable to avoid dangers to their health. At the least, they may come to depend on you, the carer, to see to their simple comforts and relief from pain, or it may be that you will be responsible for their overall safety—even their lives.

However, you are not dealing solely with the safety of your patient—there are others, as well as yourself, to consider too.

A safe and comfortable environment

Most people prefer the privacy and comfort of their own rooms when illness strikes (some aspects of this are dealt with in Chapter 12). Imagine your bedroom completely bare and stripped of all furnishing. Now build up a picture of it in your mind as you would like to have it, ideally, if you were ill. List what sort of things would be important to you. You will probably be able to identify many features which would make you feel at ease and safe and promote healing:

- Quiet room, free from loud or sudden noises—perhaps silent or with gentle background music of your choice
- Pleasant decor, flowers, plants
- Window with an open attractive view
- Comfortable bed or cot, chairs and tables of the right height

and perhaps with wheels to assist movement (but with brakes to prevent sudden movement when leaned on)
- Space enough to move around and to permit enough people with access to lift and move safely—no clutter

Many people take pills or medicine either prescribed by a doctor or bought at the chemist. If you are caring for someone, always make sure you fully understand the dose, the time the medicine or tablet is to be taken and how it works. Never give extra dosages, or omit a dose without mentioning it as soon as possible to the nurse or doctor. In addition, if you know that your patient is taking tablets from the chemist, as well as from the doctor, make sure he knows that too.

One of the most important aspects of safe practice is taking care of any medicines, including painkillers, that are prescribed for the patient. In hospital, giving of medicines is normally the function of a trained nurse, while in the home many medicines can be bought at the chemist shop or supermarket for the relief of pain. These can be given quite safely if the manufacturers' instructions are followed carefully, unless the patient is on medical treatment, when you should seek advice. Other, stronger painkillers are only available on prescription from a doctor and, again, the instructions should be followed carefully.

Medicines are best kept stored safely in a lockable cupboard, especially well away from the reach of children and always in the containers they were supplied in. In hospital, tablets and medicines should normally be handed to a trained nurse for safe custody. Keeping medicines at the bedside of adults can be dangerous too—they may awake at night and repeat a dose of drugs, forgetting that they took some recently. A disorientated person should never be left with easy access to medicines or, for that matter, other items of dangerous equipment. It is not unknown for a patient who is confused to drink from his flower vase or urinal!

In general, never help a patient to exceed the stated dose and always consult your senior nurse or doctor if the drug is not effective.

There is much that you can do to relieve pain without using drugs:

- Make sure the patient is not hungry or thirsty.
- Check that the patient's position is comfortable.
- Reduce excessive noise, heat, light or cold.
- Use suitable pillows, furniture, etc, to assist with positioning.
- Stay with the patient to reassure him or her if frightened or anxious.
- Give the patient time to express fears and anxieties and refer these difficulties to a trained person for advice if you cannot solve them.
- Offer comfort—a cuddle or holding hands can do much to relieve a person who is in pain or frightened.
- Make sure that aids are used correctly when moving the patient. Have enough people available to help, so that the patient does not overexert.
- Find out what sort of pain it is and how the patient feels it can be relieved. Report these findings to a trained nurse.
- Check with the patient that any help you have given to relieve pain is working. If not, seek advice again.

There is a lot you can do, without necessarily resorting to drugs, to promote the general comfort of someone with pain. However, always seek professional advice first if you are working in a hospital or a home under supervision.

In hospital, you may also have a responsibility for the safe keeping of valuables and clothing. There is usually a set procedure for dealing with these and you must follow it carefully, for your own benefit as well as the patient's. Another nurse should always check and record items with you—what they are and where they are stored. How you describe them also needs to be considered, for example use 'yellow metal' for gold and 'coat of fur-like type' for fur coat. There have been incidences when nurses have faced problems with the relatives or patients making inappropriate claims: (a) a patient claimed for a gold watch from the hospital (which the nurse had listed as his property) and when his valuables were returned, he argued that the watch given to him (not real gold) was not his own; (b) another patient later demanded the hospital replace a 'mink coat' (which the nurse had listed), claiming that the simulated fur coat given back to her had been substituted for her own. Legal difficulties can ensue if you are not careful, with the safe recording and custody of the patient's property.

If you work in a hospital or other such setting, it is part of your role to be fully up to date with the procedure for safety in relation to fire alert, bomb scare, major disaster, infection control and AIDS. Make sure that you attend teaching sessions on these subjects and revise the written procedures available in your area. If you don't know about the lectures or the written procedures, ask the nurse in charge. You should also ask her about the implications of the Health and Safety at Work Act and your responsibility in relation to it.

In home or hospital, we are beset by potential dangers. It is your responsibility as a carer to know what to do to prevent danger and how to act if it arises. Always act under the guidance of a trained nurse and seek advice from them when you are unsure. Report hazards promptly when you discover them and use all equipment correctly. *Keep others safe and take care of yourself too*.

Whether you are caring in home or hospital, you have a responsibility to ensure that the patient is safe and comfortable. Keep the following list in mind and, in addition, be on the look out for ways of making the patients' environment more pleasant.

- Carpets and floor surfaces that are secure, free from bumps and non-slip
- Surfaces that are clean, dust free and easy to keep clean and free from germs
- Good ventilation, draught free, comfortable temperature
- Variable lighting with effective curtains and bedside lights
- Personal items within easy reach to prevent over-reaching
- Room and occupant can be easily observed (especially if the patient is very dependent, disorientated or suicidal)
- Personal belongings and valuables can be kept safely stored
- Room easy to evacuate in case of fire or other dangers
- Furniture, etc adjusted to match limited abilities (for example blind, deaf, restricted mobility), including suitable working surfaces
- Safe energy systems, including gas fittings, electric wiring and sockets

- Medicines, cleaning agents, sharp and dangerous implements stored safely
- All equipment checked regularly for safety and used under the guidance of a trained nurse where appropriate.

The prevention of infection

Preventing the spread of infection refers as much to yourself as the patient. Dealing with the patient's personal hygiene in the general sense is dealt with in Chapter 8. In this section we examine the precautions we can take to ensure that

- Any infection that the patient may have does not spread to others
- The patient does not suffer from potential sources of infection in his or her environment
- Others do not bring infections to the patient.

We are bombarded by germs throughout our lives and most of us are able to resist serious infection because our bodies have effective ways of fighting them off. However, the risks of getting a serious infection increase if body defences are very weak (for example the very old and the very young, the malnourished or those weakened by other illnesses). We are also more at risk if we are under attack from large numbers of micro-organisms or if they are particularly virulent.

Work surfaces must be kept clean with suitable cleaning agents or disinfectants (made in the right concentrations). Laundry and other clothing must be changed regularly and promptly when soiled. Toilets, sinks and other items of personal hygiene must also be kept scrupulously clean, making sure that the equipment used for cleaning these things is not used for cleaning other items, such as cooking utensils.

Pets visiting the home can transmit infections to others and may need to be kept away from people who are very ill. It is usually quite safe, and reassuring, to let the patient's own pet be with his owner for cuddling, stroking and even sleeping, if this is what the patient is used to. Regular veterinary check-ups and treatment for worm infestations, for example, are essential, particularly with dogs and cats.

In general, people who already have infections (for example

'colds' or 'flu') should keep away from the person who is already ill, at least until they are free of infection themselves. Similarly contact by others with the patient should be kept to a minimum (especially if they are at risk because they are frail or are very small children if the patient has an infection that may spread to them). Patients with infections spread by coughing or sneezing should be encouraged to use disposable tissues, which can be removed promptly. Strict hygiene precautions and prompt disposal are needed with urine or faeces when these may be infected. When you have doubts about the likelihood of the spread of infection to or from your patient, you should consult a trained nurse or doctor for advice.

Simple wounds or scratches can be healed easily with a few precautions:

- using clean hands when changing dressings
- using a suitable antiseptic cream or lotion (as directed by the doctor or manufacturer)
- applying sterile (germ free) dressings of the type that can be bought in most chemists or stores.

Simple precautions like the above can be managed easily by yourself both at home and in hospital. If you are helping in hospital, however, you must be particularly careful to follow the directions given by the trained nurse. Not only is the ill patient more at risk, there are also more disease-producing germs in the environment. In some circumstances, special protective clothing may be needed and there may be special ways of dealing with excreta and other body fluids such as blood, vomit or sputum. As contaminated waste needs to be incinerated, and glass and sharp instruments sealed in hard containers for disposal, those caring for patients in the community must be aware of the local council's arrangements for collecting waste and soiled linen, etc.

Your own cleanliness and safety

General hygiene measures to be taken include particular attention to the cleanliness of the hands, thoroughly washing them with soap and hot water and drying on a disposable (preferably) or a clean towel. The only rings that may be worn are wedding rings. Always wash your hands before preparing food, after using the toilet, after helping your patient with his toiletting or between different patients. Nails should be kept short and nail varnish should not be worn.

Keep your own uniforms and clothing scrupulously clean. Uniforms should be kept for the hospital and not used at home. Apart from your hands, attention to your own general hygiene is very important, especially the care of your hair. If your hair is long, it needs to be kept in place, particularly when near open wounds.

If you are caring for others your services are valuable—take care of yourself too. Eat a well balanced diet and protect yourself from injury or extremes of heat or cold. Use equipment correctly (for example use the brakes on beds or furniture when moving patients) and ensure that you lift correctly, with enough people to help.

4

Mobilising

When mobilising patients, two cardinal rules apply:

- Keep your patient safe
- Keep yourself safe

Many patients have weaknesses, unsteadiness or paralysis, which necessitate help with mobilising. However, moving another body throws great strain on your own and there are correct ways of moving someone that help you to protect yourself. Your back is the site most at risk, thus it is no coincidence that back injuries are probably the most common health problem amongst nurses. You have as much responsibility to take care of yourself as you have for caring for the patient. Remember, failure to do so can render you permanently handicapped.

- Seek practical advice in lifting and moving techniques at your workplace or from the nurses or physiotherapists who are helping you care for your patient at home.
- *Never* attempt to lift or move anyone or anything after having injured your back, unless you have medical permission to do so.
- *Never* attempt to lift without first being taught and without ensuring that someone is available to help if necessary.

There are many sources of assistance to help someone who has restricted mobility. Lifting aids can be provided and assistance can be obtained for people who cannot move around without help. You need to discuss the problem with the nurse or social worker and seek their assistance if you have difficulty in establishing a claim. As well as State aid, many voluntary organisations, for example the Red Cross and St John's Ambulance Brigade, have some facilities available to help. Aids that are more easily available include chairs, sticks, walking frames and splints, whilst hand rails and stair lights can often be fitted through the local authority or another grant aiding body. Remember to ask the nurse or physiotherapist to teach both of you how to use the aid safely.

No matter how many aids you have it is essential that you always lift properly (Fig. 4.1). Find someone to help you, preferably someone who is about your height, who has also been taught how to lift. Co-ordinate your activities with careful timing and by giving clear instructions to each other. Explain carefully to the patient what you are about to do and what you want him to do. Do not rush him. Let him help as much as he is able and at his own pace. Co-ordinate your actions to his. When your patient has been safely lifted from bed to chair or from one position to another in bed make sure he is comfortable and that he can reach his table or locker.

Some good general points to remember when lifting (Fig. 4.1):

- Always lift and move your patient under the guidance of a trained nurse or physiotherapist until you feel safe and competent.

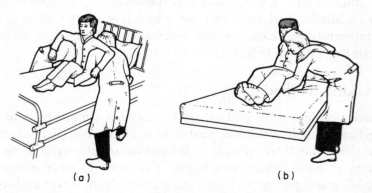

(a)   (b)

Fig. 4.1   (a) Good lift (two nurses; good posture; patient clear of bed). (b) Bad lift (one nurse; patient's skin is scraping on the bed linen, creating a shearing force; bad posture).

- Adopt the correct posture, keeping your back straight and using your bent knees for lifting and leverage. Keep your feet apart and twist your feet, not your spine, when you turn.
- Ensure that your clothing, and that of your patient, allows for ease of movement. Choose well fitting, laced, low heeled shoes with non-slip soles for both of you.
- Use lifting aids if the nurse or physiotherapist has taught you to. Check that the brakes are locked if the equipment has wheels and that the height is correct.
- Ensure that you have a clear area within which you can lift and move your patient safely.
- Position yourself and the equipment so as to minimise the amount of moving and turning required.
- Always tell your patient what you plan to do and enlist his co-operation and help.

You could ask the nurse to provide you with a copy of their staff booklet on lifting, so that you can understand why different lifts are sometimes used.

Remember:

- People . . . two
- Posture . . . good, lifting as taught
- Patient . . . helping as much as possible

It is much easier to lift a patient in a single bed that is adjusted to thigh height. If your patient is spending long periods of time being lifted in bed, or in and out of bed, it is worth talking to the community nurse concerning assistance in obtaining a hospital type bed on loan (Fig. 4.2).

Making the bed

Save yourself time and effort by using a simple bedmaking technique such as the one illustrated in Figure 4.3. Bedmaking is much quicker if two people do it together and if you have everything to hand before you begin. You need to have adequate bedding and pillows to keep your patient clean, warm and comfortable. Remember there are grants to buy bedding for the elderly and long-term sick; your nurse or social worker will be able to advise on this.

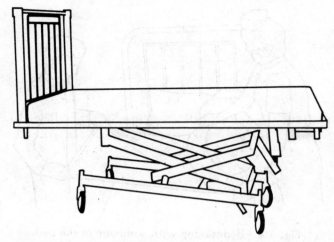

Fig. 4.2 A King's Fund bed, which may be raised and tilted and is easy to move.

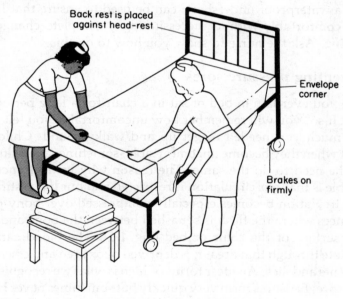

Back rest is placed against head-rest

Envelope corner

Brakes on firmly

Fig. 4.3 Bedmaking.

Bedmaking with someone in bed

It is always better to move your patient out of bed if possible. If not you should always try to have someone to help you. When

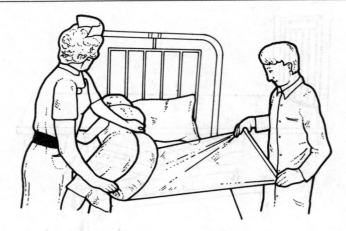

Fig. 4.4 Bedmaking with someone in the bed.

the patient is incontinent, an extra sheet (called a draw-sheet), with a waterproof undersheet, can be used to ensure that he is kept comfortable without necessitating a complete change of bedding. Ask the nurse to show you how to do this.

Preventing pressure sores

Have you ever lain in bed or sat in a chair for a long period of time? If so, you will remember how uncomfortable you felt and how much you needed to get up and walk around. Children fidget when they become uncomfortable; sometimes as adults we feel the need to do the same. The reason why we feel uncomfortable is that our circulation is restricted and our limbs stiffen. The circulation becomes especially compressed over bony prominences where the flesh is squashed between the bone and the hard surface of the chair or bed (Fig. 4.5). The blood cannot circulate through that area; it is deprived of oxygen and essential nutrients and dies. An ulcer forms, which is what we recognise as a bedsore. Bedsores form very quickly but sometimes never heal. They are very painful and are at risk of becoming infected. Long before a sore develops, the signs of poor circulation will be obvious.

The patient will complain of being uncomfortable and perhaps of having cramp. When you look at the heels, elbows and buttocks you will notice that they are red. Consequently, the

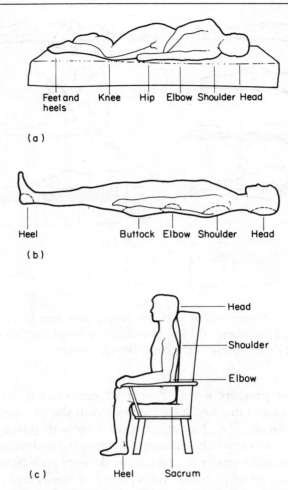

Fig. 4.5 Where pressure sores may develop: arrows indicate the 'at risk' areas. (a) Patient lying on side; (b) patient lying on back; (c) patient in chair.

patient will require help to change position and relieve pressure. Figure 4.6 shows some of the alternative positions you can use to make your patient more comfortable and to relieve that build-up of pressure which restricts the circulation and leads to bed or pressure sores. In general, patients need to be helped to change their position two-hourly (day and night).

There are many other steps you can take to relieve pressure

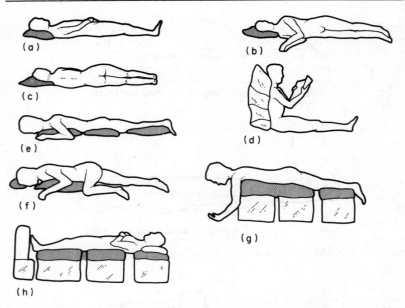

Fig. 4.6 The prevention of pressure sores: positions to be used in rotation. (a) Recumbent; (b) left lateral; (c) right lateral; (d) upright; (e) prone; (f) right lateral; (g) prone; (h) recumbent.

and prevent pressure sores. You must ensure that the bed is always clean and dry and avoid using nylon sheets which cause people to sweat. The chair must have a smooth porous cover next to the patient; when necessary, protect the bed sheet with a cotton sheet that is easily laundered. Make sure your patient eats as healthy a diet as possible, with plenty of fluids and protein. Keep the skin surfaces clean and dry, and rinse off all soap after washing. Unless your patient has been prescribed medication (lotions or powder) by the doctor, do not put anything on skin that is red or broken. The use of such things as talcum powder, methylated spirit, egg white, iodine compounds and zinc and castor oil are all known to harm even healthy skin. However, there are a number of practical aids, which you can discuss with the nurse. Some patients benefit from sitting or lying on washable sheepskins, others from using special cushions or beds; the use of wedges and splints can assist patient comfort.

It must be stressed, however, that the best way to prevent

pressure sores is to *lift* and *move* your patients as often as the nurse advises, ensuring that they are not dragged along the bed surface as they are moved.

Some patients are more at risk of developing pressure sores than others. Research has shown that those most at risk are the following:

- Frail or particularly immobile
- Emaciated or obese
- Cared for by helpers who are not lifting properly and are dragging the patient
- Those nursed on an uncomfortable surface
- Incontinent, especially if they have to wait for the bed to be changed
- Those with poor circulation, anaemia or respiratory diseases.

Other problems due to poor mobility

Bedsores are not the only potential problem of immobility. The inability to move and get about for oneself actually affects every system of the body. The list is endless:

- *Mental*: boredom, frustration, depression, loss of interest in life, feelings of hopelessness and inadequacy.
- *Social*: loss of contact with family, work and friendship activities, loss of social pleasures, often shortage of income due to unemployment.
- *Sexual*: frustration, reduced libido, effects on wife or husband, jealousy.
- *Spiritual*: difficulties in attending meetings for worship, questioning or actual loss of faith.
- *Physical*: (a) poor circulation due to lack of exercise, weakening of cardiac muscle, sluggish circulation leading to clot formation (especially in the legs and lungs), swelling of lower limbs; (b) diminished chest expansion, leading to risk of chest infections and reduced oxygen intake; (c) poor blood flow to kidneys, causing low urinary output and urinary stasis (this can cause kidney stones and urine infections); (d) muscle weakness and wastage, stiff joints, softening of bones due to shortage of calcium, contractions and deformities of limbs, foot drop, general loss of muscle tone; (e) loss of appetite,

weight loss, gastric upsets, constipation due to poor diet, immobility and an inability to use the toilet as desired; (f) general feelings of being unwell, aches, pains, headaches.

The problems of bedrest are far-reaching and most debilitating. Our aims must be twofold: to prevent, as far as possible, the complications of immobility arising and to ensure that the patient achieves the maximum degree of independence. Figures

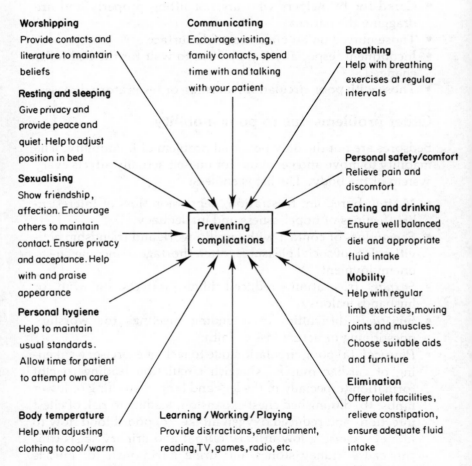

Worshipping
Provide contacts and literature to maintain beliefs

Resting and sleeping
Give privacy and provide peace and quiet. Help to adjust position in bed

Sexualising
Show friendship, affection. Encourage others to maintain contact. Ensure privacy and acceptance. Help with and praise appearance

Personal hygiene
Help to maintain usual standards. Allow time for patient to attempt own care

Body temperature
Help with adjusting clothing to cool/warm

Communicating
Encourage visiting, family contacts, spend time with and talking with your patient

Learning / Working / Playing
Provide distractions, entertainment, reading, TV, games, radio, etc.

Breathing
Help with breathing exercises at regular intervals

Personal safety/comfort
Relieve pain and discomfort

Eating and drinking
Ensure well balanced diet and appropriate fluid intake

Mobility
Help with regular limb exercises, moving joints and muscles. Choose suitable aids and furniture

Elimination
Offer toilet facilities, relieve constipation, ensure adequate fluid intake

Preventing complications

Fig. 4.7 Preventing complications: you should work with nurses and physiotherapists to achieve the following aims (bold). See the relevant chapters for more details.

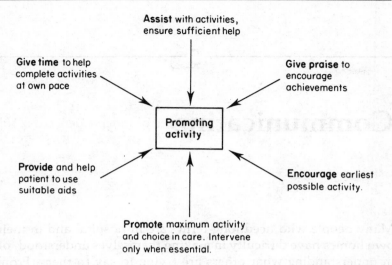

Fig. 4.8 Promoting activities: you should work with physiotherapists, occupational therapists and nurses to plan activities.

4.7 and 4.8 outline the factors associated with these aims, and in both cases the nursing *goal* is positioned in the centre, and the nursing *actions* highlighted around the edges. No one person can do all this alone. You will require the help of friends and family as well as professional carers if you are going to achieve such nursing goals.

Finally, try to imagine what it feels like to have a mobility problem and to be dependent on others. Imagine you are confined to bed in one room, with an illness that has already lasted two to three weeks and from which you are now slowly recovering. Write down how you think you are feeling and how the illness is affecting your lifestyle.

Being immobile forces dependency on us. The person who is caring for someone with a mobility problem needs great skill and patience in order to prevent the patient from becoming distressed at being a 'burden'. Remember to ask for help from other people, the nurse, your doctor and relations, so that you yourself don't become overtired or ill.

5

Communicating

Many people who need long-term care in hospital and in their own homes have difficulty in making themselves understood, or in understanding what others are trying to say to them. From before birth human beings are conditioned to respond to voices and noises. Any mother knows how a loud or sudden noise will startle a sleeping baby just as she knows that her voice will quieten her child quicker than anyone else's voice.

Hearing

Hearing is the first sense that develops; by listening to and then copying all the sounds he hears the child learns to speak. Then he can both understand and be understood.

Deafness is an invisible handicap and even severe deafness can remain undetected for many months. The deaf child may be described as 'slow', 'backward' or 'withdrawn'. The same withdrawal is evident in the person of any age who becomes deaf and the deafness isolates the person from the community he lives within. The prime communication sense is gone; he can no longer hear what is being said, listen to music or the radio, or enjoy the simple things of life like the sound of his cat purring. He cannot hear the doorbell, and the telephone—often the lifeline for the person living alone—becomes useless.

Do not simply imagine what it would be like; go to your chemist and buy some wax earplugs. Keep them in all the evening and realise just what you miss when you are deaf. You cannot hear your children's tales of the day at school, the train announcement at the station or the kettle whistling. Have you ever turned the sound down on the television? Or listened to the sound and compared the sound with the sub-titles when they appear? How much of the storyline would you miss?

Caring for those who are deaf or partially deaf can be as frustrating for the carer as it is for the deaf person. If you can appreciate how the deafness occurs it can help you plan care to assist constructively.

Sound waves enter the outer ear (Fig. 5.1) and pass to the tympanic membrane. The membrane vibrates and the sound waves are passed across the middle ear to the window, which also vibrates. This vibration causes small hairs inside the inner ear to vibrate and it is this vibration which triggers the nerve endings in the inner ear. Nervous impulses are then sent to the brain for interpretation.

A blockage anywhere along this pathway can cause

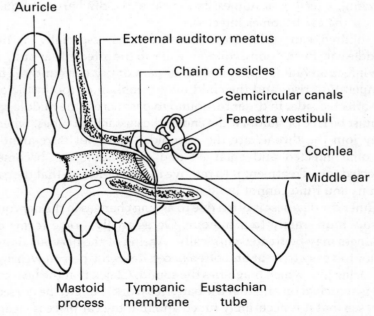

Fig. 5.1 The ear. From Jackson S.M. and Bennett P.J. (1988) *Physiology with anatomy for nurses*. London: Baillière Tindall.

conductive deafness and is by far the most common cause of hearing loss. Far rarer is neural deafness, in which the nervous tissue itself is damaged.

Many elderly people expect to lose some hearing as they age. Although ageing changes can cause deafness, the first thing the GP will do is check the outer ear for wax build-up and arrange for his patient to receive a NHS hearing test if he suspects the problem is more serious. Wax can be removed by simple syringing carried out by a doctor or nurse. Prior to syringing the patient may be advised to instill drops into the ears so that the wax can be softened. Following syringing, antibiotic drops may be prescribed if there is any sign of infection.

You may be asked to help someone instill prescribed drops, or to advise them how to do it themselves. The nurse in charge will teach you how to do this. Once you know that someone has had to have their ears syringed you can watch out for the wax build-up to occur again and let the sister or doctor know. As wax builds up in the outer ear people experience a gradual hearing loss, buzzing, a feeling of fullness in the ear and a discharge of liquid wax if the ear becomes infected.

Children can suffer from ear infections, especially in the middle ear. Even young children will rub the affected ear and, as the infection builds up, complain of pain or cry constantly. The temperature rises and the child may complain of toothache on the affected side. In order for sound to pass across the middle ear it must be free of fluid. At the end of the eustachian tubes, where they join the throat, are the adenoids; these not infrequently become infected and enlarged and the middle ear becomes infected too. Treatment is to remove the adenoids, so that the ear drains and fluid cannot build up again.

Inner ear deafness is often due to ageing changes in the nervous tissue, more rarely to a tumour. Occasionally, some forms of deafness may be treated surgically. Ageing of the nervous tissue is not too easy to treat and often necessitates the person wearing a hearing aid, which magnifies the sound. Check that the hearing aid is switched on and that the batteries work. Fit it to the correct ear, see that it is accurately tuned and that the ear piece is clean.

When talking with anyone who has a hearing problem sit or stand at their level and face them. Speak distinctly (not necessarily slowly and certainly not in 'simple terms'), moving your lips correctly. Do not slur your words and do not use slang expressions or abbreviations. Use your hands to assist in describing what you are saying and you may find a pencil and paper helpful in ensuring that instructions are understood. Try not to raise your voice. This does not help and only serves to enable everyone else to hear the conversation as well. If the person has a hearing aid, check that it is correctly tuned and try speaking into it.

It is even more difficult to communicate with someone who does not speak English as a first language. As well as trying to hear what is being said, the listener may also have to translate inside his head. This is when you will need your pencil and paper and will need to use your hands. It may help if you ask if you can discuss the instructions with a relative or friend so that they can reinforce the information.

If normal conversation is difficult, the Red Cross can provide cards in English and many other languages. Some hospitals and other charities provide booklets which can assist everyone, not only the deaf.

Always remember the basic rules of talking. Take your time, seem interested in the conversation, smile, look in the person's eyes and give him or her time to answer. All these non-verbal signs of communication are as essential to understanding as clear speech.

When speaking with the visually handicapped person we need to consider other methods of non-verbal communication.

Seeing

Visual failing is much more common than deafness and happens to most of us as we age. In many instances it can be quickly and easily corrected by spectacles. In April 1989 a charge of £10 will be introduced for eye tests. However, tests will remain free of charge to children, elderly citizens and students under 19 years of age. Assistance is often available for the purchase of glasses or magnifying lenses; the nurse or social worker will advise.

As with the ear, if you understand how the eye works it can

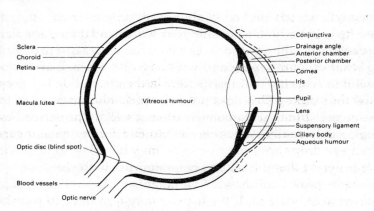

Conjunctiva
Sclera
Drainage angle
Choroid
Anterior chamber
Retina
Posterior chamber
Cornea
Iris
Macula lutea
Vitreous humour
Pupil
Lens
Suspensory ligament
Ciliary body
Aqueous humour
Optic disc (blind spot)
Blood vessels
Optic nerve

Fig. 5.2 The eye. From Jackson S.M. and Bennett P.J. (1988) *Physiology with anatomy for nurses*. London: Baillière Tindall.

help you to appreciate the problems that patients experience and why (Fig. 5.2).

Light rays enter the eye through the clear cornea, pass through the pupil, across the lens and into the retinal nerve endings. The lens has the power to alter shape (focus) so that the light rays fall on the most sensitive part of the retina. In the retina the nerve endings convert the light rays into nervous impulses, which pass along the optic nerve for interpretation by the brain. This is known as the visual pathway. In order for the light rays to pass smoothly along the pathway the cornea and lens must be clear and the nervous tissue healthy.

The common problem occurs due to ageing changes in the lens, which become less elastic as we get older, so that one needs to wear glasses to help the focusing power of the lens, ensuring that light falls on the retina. Some people need to wear glasses from an early age because the lens loses this ability earlier than in middle age.

However, as one approaches later middle age and old age as many as one in eight of us will develop a cataract. Cataracts occur because the lens loses its clarity. Cataracts occasionally occur in children due to congenital disease and as a result of injury to the eye or because the person has diabetes that is unstable (see Chapter 10). The cloudy lens no longer transmits the light rays, the patient's vision gradually gets more cloudy and eventually the person cannot see. Then the lens must be removed surgically.

The other common ageing condition which affects the vision is glaucoma. This is due to a blockage in the circulation in the eye and if the blockage is not removed nerve damage occurs and the person goes blind. Treatment is often given by prescribed eye drops; occasionally surgery is used to effect a permanent cure. When eye drops are prescribed you may be asked to help with administering them; a registered nurse will advise you.

Whatever the cause the partially sighted and blind person has problems in making him/herself understood or in understanding. They cannot see who they are talking to, interpret facial expressions or make eye contact. In addition, because loss of sight affects mobility, they become socially isolated as well. If they belong to a community which uses hands to support speech (Italian, French, for example), they have further problems. Try putting cotton pads over your eyes for a few hours and discover how this affects your communication.

Most people who experience visual disturbance consult their optician. He will prescribe glasses and refer the patient to their GP if further help is needed. Once obtained the glasses must be kept clean and checked occasionally to ensure that they fit correctly. Replacement testing is advised every two years. If two pairs of glasses are needed, advise that the frames should be different so that the user can tell which is which. When not in use they should be stored in a case or kept lens side uppermost in a safe place. The practice of a chain around the neck can be useful but care must be taken not to scratch the lenses as this distorts vision.

Simple eye infections are common in children, the elderly and the ill person. Advise your patient to consult his or her GP and not to treat it him/herself.

As vision deteriorates, people become increasingly dependent on sound and touch. Always announce your presence before you get too close and touch the person. 'Hello! It's Susan and I've brought your lunch' is so much friendlier than putting the plate noisily down in front of someone who was not expecting it. Remember to explain what is on the plate and to ask if further assistance is needed with cutting food. Put drinks within reach, explaining where they are placed so that they are not knocked over. Verbal explanation is all the more important when one cannot see clearly and after imparting information always confirm understanding.

Try to encourage your partially sighted person to care for himself as much as possible. A telephone is a great aid to independence. In some families, especially when there is a child involved, or where the community cares very well for its aged relatives (i.e. Indian or Pakistani patients) there is a tendency for the blind person to be totally cared for. Try to explain how essential it is for self-esteem that the person does as much as possible for himself.

Voluntary organisations can offer considerable assistance to the blind and partially sighted patient, which can help them to remain in contact with day to day activities. The Royal National Institute for the Blind (RNIB), as well as local libraries, can provide talking books and large print reading material; there is a Braille Radio Times available each week for radio listeners. Magnifying glasses can also be used to ensure that maximum use is made of all remaining sight.

Speaking

Perhaps one of our most basic communicating senses is that of speech. Sadly, those born deaf may never acquire clear speech since speech develops in association with sound interpretation. Often such children become very skilled in sign language and other non-verbal communication and, through considerable effort, may make themselves understood.

Those who lose speech later in life experience considerable psychological and social trauma. Their most active communication asset is gone. The most common reason for sudden loss of speech is a stroke. Fortunately, time is a great healer and with effort and assistance from a speech therapist, speech often returns. Initially though, there is a great sense of frustration, especially since the patient knows what he wants to say but cannot 'get it out'. Strokes also affect other areas of the brain concerned with speech; nowhere is this more traumatic than when a patient has learnt English as a second language, and the memory centre is affected. For example imagine that your family and friends only speak English and all you can remember is the Ukrainian from your childhood.

It is difficult to learn to speak again without perseverance and skilled therapy but one can do much to assist. If the patient has dentures, make sure that they are in place and fitting correctly; sit at your patient's level and allow him time to talk; do not hurry him by finishing sentences, especially as this increases misunderstandings. It may be useful to ask questions, especially if these require 'yes/no' answers. However, remember some people will answer what they think you want to hear. Use aids if they help—like the Red Cross language cards—and remember to respect that patient's privacy.

Touch and smell

When we talk about communication we often forget the other two senses: touch and smell. Perhaps this is because they are little used in day to day communication. However, both are important since both allow us to express our feelings and they assume greater importance when one or another communication sense is impaired.

Human sense of smell is not highly developed and yet we can all recognise the perfume a loved one wears, or smell alcohol or garlic on the breath. Acetone on the breath of a diabetic warns the carer to review diet and drug regimen and to discuss stabilisation with the nurse or doctor, whilst the smell of bad teeth will indicate the need for a dental review or be a percursor of general ill health. It is important that the carer smells clean and fresh. No uniforms or cardigans stained with sweat, no heady perfume and no scented make-up. Remember your patient may like to smell nice too, so offer talcum powder and after-shave after washing or shaving.

It is equally important not to show distaste for your patient's body smells. Instead, do everything possible to assist in coping with the problem (whether they see it as a problem or not). Colostomies rarely smell if properly protected by an appliance that fits but to wrinkle one's nose up is bad mannered and uncaring. Mention the smell to the nurse so that she can advise on a change of appliance or the use of a deodoriser. Remember that smells you find offensive (smoke, alcohol, garlic) may not be offensive to the patient so be careful just how you discuss 'smelly' problems.

Just as it might take direct action to 'face' a smell front without showing distaste or displeasure, you may have to touch someone with a skin infection or infestation. One of the best ways of showing we care is to touch one another; to hold their arm or shake their hand. Remember that provided you observe basic hygiene rules, few skin rashes are infectious, and fleas and nits jump only a few inches. If you are in contact with an infested patient, ask the nurse or doctor for advice on how to shampoo and wash.

Communication is an integral part of caring and one which we need to work at to do well. However, the effort brings its own rewards in the prevention of loneliness, isolation and social loss. This chapter aims to help you to care for patients who are experiencing diminishing loss of one or more senses for one reason or another. The care of the totally blind, deaf or aphasic (one who cannot speak) person needs very skilled 'advice and care' and you should be specially prepared to give this if necessary.

6

Breathing

You may recall the story of the spoiled child who, when she could not get her way, threatened to hold her breath until she died: she did not succeed. Our breathing is normally controlled automatically by the brain (it monitors the blood for the levels of oxygen and carbon dioxide present) to reduce or increase our breathing according to the body's need for oxygen.

Taking in oxygen and getting rid of the waste product carbon dioxide are the primary reasons for breathing. To some extent we can control our breathing, speeding it up, interrupting it or slowing it down at will. Some people (for example experienced divers) can hold their breath for three or four minutes but most of us begin to feel uncomfortable after a minute or two and very soon the desire to breathe again is overwhelming.

We breathe to live; if we are deprived of oxygen for more than a few minutes our lives are at risk. The oxygen is transported in the bloodstream. Anything that prevents oxygen getting into the lungs and across into the blood or, for that matter, anything that prevents the blood flowing easily (such as the reduced pumping action of a diseased heart) can seriously affect our health. Some parts of our bodies can be deprived of oxygen for quite long periods (for example severed limbs have been restored to bodies with considerable success in recent years), while other parts are very sensitive to oxygen deprivation. The brain is particularly delicate in this respect: if suddenly deprived of oxygen for more than two or three minutes (by strangulation, for example) it rapidly 'shuts down', rendering us unconscious. Any longer than

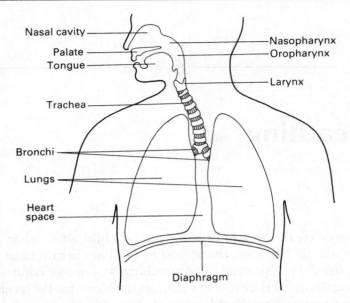

Nasal cavity

Palate

Tongue

Trachea

Bronchi

Lungs

Heart
space

Nasopharynx

Oropharynx

Larynx

Diaphragm

Fig. 6.1   The respiratory tract. From Jackson S.M. and Bennett P.J. (1988) *Physiology with anatomy for nurses*. London: Baillière Tindall.

this and brain cells begin to die, resulting in worsening brain damage and eventually death.

Apnoea

One rise and fall of the chest (as the chest muscles contract and relax) is *one respiration*, and most adults at rest do this about 15–20 times each minute. Timing these respirations each minute gives us the *respiratory rate*. Try checking the respiratory rate on a few friends and note the differences. Select people of varying ages. You will find that babies may breathe at over 40 respirations per minute, a child of 10 or 11 years at 25–30 respirations per minute. Heavy smoking adults and those with chest diseases will tend to breathe much faster than average. Breathing rates are less when sleeping and higher when we are excited or when exercising. You may obtain a false reading if someone knows their breathing is being counted.

Cessation of breathing (apnoea) leading to lack of oxygen to the brain (cerebral anoxia) is therefore potentially fatal and must be recognised for what it is—an emergency. It can arise as a result of disease processes in the lungs, for example, or as a result of blockages of the air passages (asphyxia). The colour of the patient's skin changes rapidly: a 'blueness' (cyanosis) is noted, affecting the lips, ears, toes and fingertips most markedly at first, then quickly affecting the whole appearance. The rise and fall of the chest and the gentle movements of the abdomen associated with breathing come to a halt. If conscious at first, the patient will become extremely frightened and restless, struggling to cough, gasping and clutching at the neck.

Emergency care: artificial respiration

If not relieved, the patient will rapidly become unconscious. It becomes increasingly difficult to revive (resuscitate) the patient as more time passes, leading to irreversible brain damage and then death.

In such an emergency the following rules apply:

- Know the procedure to follow in your place of work if you suspect a patient has stopped breathing and give alert assistance to the experts as they request it during the resuscitation.
- If you suspect that someone has stopped breathing get help quickly, either by calling or by sounding an alarm button. If in doubt, *act* (better safe than sorry).
- Prevent obstruction of the patient's airway in the first place, particularly if he is at risk (for example if he is unconscious). The neck should be kept extended to prevent the tongue from blocking the air passage (Figs 6.2 and 6.3). Become an expert in the maintenance of a clear airway.
- Follow the procedure outlined in Figures 6.4 and 6.5. In order to feel confident, seek advice from the experts: join a first aid class. Many deaths could be prevented if everyone learned the first aid techniques necessary for clearing the airway and administering artificial respiration.
- Once the patient has resumed breathing, the airway can be kept open with your hand by correct positioning of the head until help arrives. If the patient's body is placed in the recovery

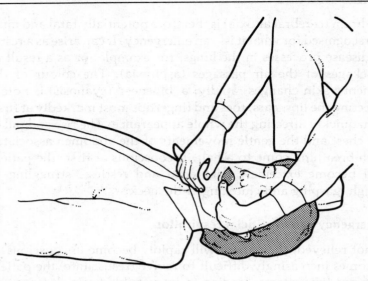

Fig. 6.2 Lay patient on back, clear any obstruction from mouth and turn head upwards.

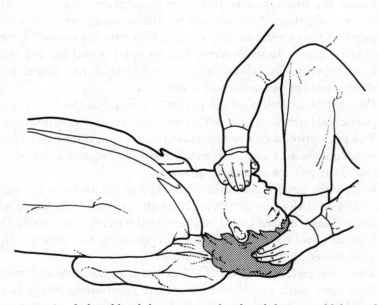

Fig. 6.3 Angle head back by pressing forehead down and lifting chin up.

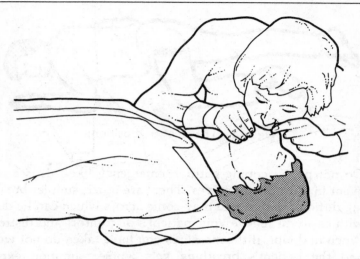

Fig. 6.4 Blow gently into patient's mouth until the chest rises; then remove your mouth.

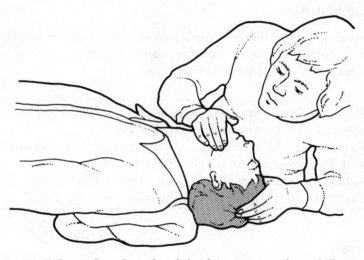

Fig. 6.5 Take a deep breath while the patient's chest deflates and repeat blowing procedure until breathing starts or help arrives.

position (Fig. 6.6), the airway will also be kept clear of the tongue, while at the same time allowing any excess saliva or vomit to drain out of the patient's mouth and not be inhaled.

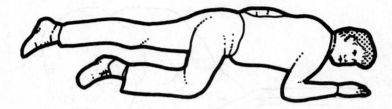

Fig. 6.6   The recovery position.

- Do not panic: coping with an emergency like this is a rare event in most people's lives. There are other, simpler breathing difficulties that you may come across which can be dealt with easily to relieve your patient's discomfort and distress. When in doubt, if the measures you have taken do not work and the patient's breathing gets worse, summon expert medical or nursing help.

Case histories

To examine some of these simple techniques, let us consider three case histories. Think about each example carefully and make a few notes on what you might do to help.

Patient 1: Emma, a young woman with a 'cold'—her nose is blocked and her throat swollen and sore.
Patient 2: Matthew, a child having an 'asthma' attack—frightened and 'fighting for his breath'.
Patient 3: Jack, an elderly man with a chest infection, struggling to breathe and coughing up thick sputum.

Emma

Much relief can be given to a sore throat without resort to medicines. Many people find ice-cream or sips of cold or iced drinks particularly soothing. Lozenges can be purchased and many proprietary gargles are available from your chemist (follow the directions for use carefully) while the old-fashioned salt and water gargle (one teaspoon of salt to a cupful of warm water) several times a day can be just as effective. Help is more effective if it is given kindly and sympathetically: Emma should be given time to take the treatments at her own pace and the gargle should be removed promptly after use if she could not get to the bathroom to manage the procedure herself. If in hospital, you will have to follow procedures set by the trained nurse; giving medicines is always supervised in this way.

An inhalation might also be helpful. Hospitals usually have set procedures to follow. At home, a simple method can easily be adapted. A jug of hot water (steaming but not boiling) placed in a separate bowl to steady it can be used with a suitable additive (for example menthol) to the water. A towel could be draped over Emma's head while she breathes in the vapours—in through the nose and out through the mouth for about 15 minutes. Tissues or hankerchiefs for her to blow her nose need to be available.

Warning: make sure the inhalation is on a firm surface and stay to support and supervise the patient, especially if she is weak or restless. At all times Emma will need to rest and keep warm, preferably in bed or a comfortable chair.

Matthew

Matthew will need comfort and reassurance. All breathing problems can be frightening and fear only aggravates the patient's difficulties. Provide tissues onto which Matthew can cough out any sputum and help him to take any special drugs as prescribed by the doctor. Remove any tight clothing from around the neck and chest and suggest that he will find breathing much easier sitting upright, perhaps with a table in front of him to lean on. The effort of breathing could make him hot and sweaty and a gentle wash during and after the attack can be very soothing. Whether at home or hospital, Matthew would be reassured to know that there is always someone in easy reach: a call bell or button could be placed nearby. Many patients who have had asthma for a long time become expert at managing their own problem and usually feel more secure if they know their medicines are always near at hand. Where it is related to an allergy, the source needs to be identified and avoided.

Jack

Jack will find the effort of breathing very tiring. All the things he needs should be in easy reach so that he does not waste energy trying to get them. Tissues or a sputum pot should be nearby and a drink easily available. (People with breathing difficulties breathe more through the mouth, making it very dry. Normally we breathe through the nose which moistens the air as we inhale.)

It will be particularly important for Jack to adopt a position that helps him to expand his chest easily. Remove tight clothing and again a wash will reduce sweating and discomfort associated with laboured breathing. Jack should sit upright, —either in bed or a chair, and will find well placed pillows a source of support (placed like a wedge behind his back so that his chest and shoulders can move freely). Leaning forward on a table for support (perhaps with a pillow under his arms to relieve pressure on his elbows) will also permit greater freedom for chest expansion. A pillow or board at the bottom of the bed to rest his feet on will prevent him slipping down the bed. A warm but well ventilated room is essential. You may be asked to note any changes in his breathing pattern or the colour of his sputum and report them to the doctor. A clean cream carton can be used if no sputum pot is available and tissues need to be supplied. Sputum is a source of infection and you should dispose of it promptly (preferably sealing pots in a bag and burning them), avoiding contact with your hands and washing them afterwards.

The above three case histories will help you to understand the many simple ways you can help someone with breathing difficulties. However, it must be reiterated that you should seek advice if the breathing does not improve or gets worse.

Other difficulties with breathing

Halitosis (bad breath)

Halitosis usually occurs because of increased bacterial activity in the mouth, for example with dental caries (bad teeth) or the general debility of other illness. Help with good dental hygiene or mouthwashes can improve the problem and the cause needs to be identified and dealt with. Plenty of drinks, especially fresh fruit juices, and avoiding smoking are also helpful.

Epistaxis

Epistaxis is bleeding from the nose. It may occur for no apparent reason or be associated with violent sneezing, trauma or more serious illnesses. It can be simply treated by sitting the patient upright, head forward slightly (so that blood is not swallowed), and by pinching the nose firmly under the bridge. A cold compress (for example a cloth containing ice cubes) may also be helpful if applied to the nose. Persistent or severe bleeding requires urgent medical attention.

Haemoptysis

Haemoptysis is coughing up of blood and should always be reported to a doctor for investigation. Both this and epistaxis can be very frightening events for patients and they need not only your practical help, but reassurance that you are dealing with the matter promptly and getting expert help and advice.

Tracheostomy

Tracheostomy is an artificial hole made in the trachea (the windpipe) in the lower part of the neck. It may be temporary or permanent and is usually put in place to relieve any obstruction in the windpipe higher up. A tube, often of metal or plastic, is inserted to keep the tracheostomy open. Caring for this tube in hospital is normally the province of the trained nurse. You should be aware that most patients with these tubes are unable to speak to or call you (have call bells and pen and paper nearby). Patients with permanent tracheostomies are taught to care for them themselves and you may need to help with cleaning the tube to prevent blockage with sputum. It can be rinsed in running water and a mild antiseptic. A tube is usually no longer necessary when the tracheostomy is well established.

Oxygen therapy

Again this is a procedure normally managed by a trained nurse in hospital but occasionally you may be helping a patient who is dealing with this himself at home. In hospital oxygen may be piped through wall-mounted fittings; it is stored in cylinders (black and white). It is passed through a valve which controls the flow via a mask and tubes to the patient. The doctor will prescribe the correct rate of flow and this must be followed exactly. Oxygen is necessary for life but it can also be dangerous to some patients if taken in much higher quantities than normal. When given for long periods it is best passed through a humidifier as concentrated oxygen is very drying to the mouth.

Where oxygen is in use no flames or smoking are allowed because of the fire risk.

Cough

Coughing is a way of clearing secretions from the chest and throat. When constant, it can be very tiring and disturbing for the patient. Inhalation as described above may soothe a dry cough and medicines can be given as prescribed by the doctor. You may be asked to help nurses and physiotherapists to help the patient with coughing and breathing exercises to clear the chest. A dry unproductive cough can be eased with simple linctuses; once sputum is being produced then help with removal of secretion, as described above, is needed.

Smoking

Smoking not only creates illness but makes others worse, particularly breathing difficulties. Under these circumstances it should be reduced to an absolute minimum or given up altogether. If you are a smoker yourself, you should not smoke in the presence of someone with a breathing difficulty.

Hiccups

The diaphragm (a large muscle at the base of the chest, separating it from the abdomen) may go into spasm, producing hiccups.

Sometimes the well known remedies, such as breathing in and out of a paper bag, may help but the condition may subside of its own accord after a short time. When persistent a doctor's advice should be sought.

Conclusion

Remember failure to breath comfortably and to obtain enough oxygen to maintain life is frightening because it is life-threatening. If your patient consistently has a problem and simple remedies or the prescribed medical treatment are not relieving the problem consult your nurse or the patient's GP. Make sure they know about the breathing problem so that steps can be taken to alleviate it.

Eating, drinking and eliminating

Ensuring that those we care for eat correctly is important. Many people, especially the young, the old and those who live alone do not eat well. The ill are even less likely to eat well unless someone else assists them at every stage: buying, preparing, cooking, perhaps even eating and eliminating.

Food is needed to supply energy for the activities of daily living, for the quality and repair of body tissues (bones, teeth) and for the functioning of body processes (without adequate glucose in our diets brain cell function is impaired.)

A healthy diet

A healthy diet includes a combination of proteins (found in meat and vegetables), carbohydrates (bread, milk), fats (again found in meat, dairy produce and any oily food) and water. The amount of each substance needed to maintain a healthy diet depends on age. A teenager needs considerably more of all food substances (especially protein and carbohydrate) than does the office worker. Each day the individual needs to eat a balanced diet composed of meat, dairy produce, vegetables and bread, accompanied by clear fluid. These foods will ensure that adequate vitamins and nutrients are ingested, thereby avoiding deficiency diseases.

Carbohydrates are found in fruit, sugary foods, milk, bread, grains and, in small amounts, meat and vegetables.

Fats are found in dairy produce, meat, oily foods and some vegetables.

Proteins are found in meat, fish, dairy produce (especially cheese), eggs, vegetables, bread and pulses.

The *Minerals* we need are easily eaten if the diet is healthy. Calcium for bone and tooth growth is found in dairy produce and green vegetables. Iron (for healthy blood and consequently energy) is found in meat, green vegetables and egg yolks. These are the most important nutrients but we also need potassium, iodine, copper, fluoride and others to maintain a healthy body.

Vitamins are needed in the body only in small amounts but correct growth and development is impossible without an adequate intake. Vitamins also help us to maintain health. They may be prescribed by a doctor, many vitamins contain minerals too and can be given to a patient who needs a supplementary supply.

- Vitamin A is found in red meat, egg yolk and green vegetables and helps to prevent infection as well as influencing growth.
- Vitamin D is found in milk and added to some cereals and margarines. It is essential to the growth and preservation of bones and teeth.
- Vitamin E is present in minute amounts in most foods, especially vegetables. It is essential to red blood cell production and treatment of wounds.
- Vitamin K is also found in green vegetables and red meat and it too plays a part in the healing process.
- Vitamin B is present in cereals and meat and maintains nervous tissue and digestion. It is needed in larger amounts in pregnancy and whilst the mother is breast-feeding.

A healthy diet containing adequate amounts of all these foodstuffs is essential to healthy life and carers are often asked to advise patients and relatives on appropriate diets, especially if the patient is not eating well. The nurse or doctor will be only too happy to advise on diet and to refer the patient to a dietician if necessary. It is important that any dietary advice considers patient's cultural, religious or social practices. Your health authority will have guidelines to help you care better for patients from other countries or those whose religious practices restrict

what they can eat. Advice is usually available concerning vege-
tarian diets too.

Social habits also affect eating. Most people enjoy preparing
food to share with others and enjoy the company of friends and
relatives whilst they eat. Cooking and eating alone is never as
pleasant and many people who have to do this tend to live off
soup, sandwiches and other convenience foods. This encourages
nutritional deficiencies and is one reason why successive British
governments have supported the free school meals service,
Meals on Wheels and luncheon clubs.

As well as eating a balanced diet, dieticians recommend
regular meals. This is especially important for children and the
elderly since they need to maintain a constant level of nutrition
for energy and warmth. Doctors, nurses and dieticians constantly emphasise the need to eat breakfast to provide necessary
energy to start the day.

Other carers are asked to advise on purchasing, preparing,
serving and storing foods. It is useful to know which shops and
supermarkets will sell small portions—suitable for one
person—and to be able to advise on cuts of meat and fish that are
attractive in small quantities. There are also many alternative
foods that provide adequate nutrients (cheese and eggs, for
example), which can be suggested to those who wish to reduce
meat consumption and who are looking for cheaper meals.
When considering what to recommend the preparation time and
methods used for cooking need to be taken into account. The
tougher cuts of meat require longer and slower cooking times
and are unsuitable for those who need to prepare meals in a
hurry. Many older people are unsure of new methods of
cooking—like microwave ovens and slow cookers—even when
they possess them, and may need encouraging to use them. If
food is being prepared for a family or a group of people, individual preferences have to be considered. It may prove possible to
steam fish for the patient who needs food that is easily digestible,
whilst frying it for other family members.

Preparation of food

How to clean food, whether or not to peel it and how long it can
be kept, are questions we all have to ask each time we shop and

cook. Most foods now have a recommended 'eat by' date. Food that is stored for too long may not only harm the eater but will certainly lose some of its nutritional value, as well as taste and possibly colour.

Although there an increasing number of people eating fibre in their diets and achieving this by not peeling vegetables and fruit, other people find this unacceptable. It may be more acceptable to increase fibre by the use of porridge, cereals and fibre-enriched white bread (rather than wholemeal brown).

Older people also tend to overcook vegetables, thereby reducing nutrient and fibre value, and need encouragement to change this practice and to include other fibre-rich sources in their diets.

Presentation of food

The serving of food is also important if patients are to be encouraged to eat. We have already seen that people eat better with friends, so encourage your patient to eat with others where possible. If the patient lives alone, other ways can be used to make meals attractive: leave the tray attractively set, so that all the patient needs to do is to add the food; put a single flower on the tray or table; make sure the cutlery and crockery is clean and matches, and the glass shines—these all help. If your patient needs to have food prepared in advance (for example soup which is left in a thermos), you can vary the soup, making sure that if it has to be taken from a cup not a bowl it is not lumpy. Make sure sandwiches that are left for eating later on are wrapped in clingfilm or greaseproof paper or placed in an airtight tin and are quartered as appropriate. Fruit, except for banana, can also be kept in foil. Do not forget that, if your patient does not possess a fridge, assistance is available from the social worker or the DSS. (Assistance is also available for the purchase of a cooker.)

Serve small portions if you know a larger meal will be left uneaten and leave biscuits and milk or homemade cake and a milky drink available for later. Ensure that your patient has some means of washing his or her hands before eating; alcohol- or spirit-impregnated wipes are useful if he or she cannot reach a wash basin unaided. Gastric infection can only be prevented if hygiene rules are observed.

Remember that if you are worried about a patient's or relative's diet ask the nurse, health visitor or doctor for advice. There is a wide range of diet supplements available and some of these may be acceptable instead of a main meal or before retiring to bed.

Health considerations

If there is no health reason why your patient is not managing to eat a normal diet, it may be advisable to make one or two checks. Ensure that he or she can use a knife, fork or spoon. Often patients with advanced arthritis or rheumatism need special equipment (see page 178 for list of addresses); they may also need specially adapted crockery.

Check that dentures fit and arrange a dental visit if they are uncomfortable. Ill fitting dentures are one reason why mouth infections or ulcers develop, and digestion and swallowing difficulties can also make meals unattractive. Eating loses its appeal if you know that you will suffer for it hours afterwards! People who suffer with swallowing or digestive difficulties do not always need to consult their doctor. They may need to avoid rich foods, fatty foods, fried foods and raw vegetables and fruit, since these foods are known to predispose to digestive difficulties. It may also help if food is mashed, minced or stewed.

Case histories

Consider the different dietary needs of the following two patients, both of whom have to have a lunchtime tray left by a relative.

Sally is 42 and married with sons at secondary school. She was injured in a road accident some years ago and spends her day in a wheelchair. The kitchen in her bungalow is too small for her to move around easily in her chair so her husband leaves her a lunch on a tray in the lounge and she eats a full meal with her family at 6 p.m. She is prone to put on weight and, like many immobile patients, is likely to be constipated.

Jack is an 81 year old pensioner who lives with his daughter and son-in-law. He is active and enjoys gardening and reading but has never cooked. He likes his daughter to leave him something 'easy' for lunch and, like Sally, has his main meal in the evening.

Both patients could enjoy soup, sandwiches and fruit or yoghurt. However, in Sally's case, you may wish to use a 'slimline' or diet soup, whilst if Jack is underweight or has a small appetite, the calorie content can be increased by adding cream. Similarly, although both like high-fibre bread, you would use a low-calorie spread on Sally's sandwiches. Both should eat fruit with the skin on, but you need to ensure that Jack is able to chew. Leave a suitable drink, a napkin and something for Sally to wash her hands with.

Fluid intake

Remember that many people like a drink of water with a meal and tea or coffee afterwards. Unless the doctor or nurse advises against it, sharing a glass of wine can stimulate the appetite and some beers, particularly stout, have nutritional value. Older people especially may like a warm drink before retiring and some take a tot of brandy or whisky. This can aid sleep and is a natural alternative to sleeping drugs, which can leave one drowsy and confused the next day.

People who do not drink enough can become confused, due to dehydration. They are also prone to urinary infection and constipation. Patients should be discouraged from drinking less because they have to get up in the night or because they fear bed-wetting. If they develop a urine infection they are much more likely to have a disturbed night.

Elimination of waste products

Everything that we eat or drink is processed in the body into substances for cell growth and replacement. Waste material must be eliminated. After being chemically churned up in the stomach with various gastric juices, the food passes into the small intestine for further juices to act upon it. In the small intestine all essential components, such as protein, carbohydrates, fats, vitamins and minerals, are absorbed into the bloodstream, leaving the waste products. These pass into the large intestine (colon), where water is removed, leaving formed faeces. The faeces move along the colon into the rectum by intermittent muscular contractions and relaxations known as peristalsis. In

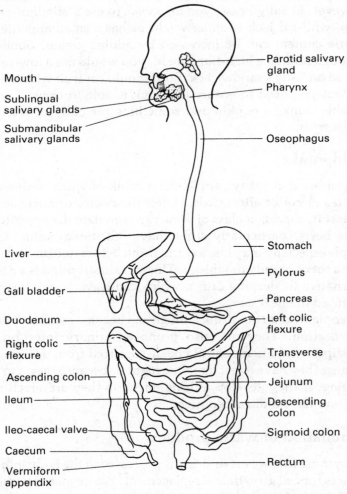

Fig. 7.1 The alimentary system. From Jackson S.M. and Bennett P.J. (1988) *Physiology with anatomy for nurses*. London: Baillière Tindall.

the rectum the faeces are stored until we are able to void them at the appropriate time in the appropriate place. The final muscles in the alimentary tract are those of the anus which are a group of muscles under voluntary control.

Blood takes essential nutrients to all the cells in the body and picks up all waste products; these are known as the waste products of metabolism, for example urea. The blood therefore also needs to get rid of these unwanted products. This is carried out by the kidneys, which filter the blood and in so doing produce urine (Fig. 7.2) The urine carries the waste products from the kidneys via the ureters to the bladder. The bladder is the reservoir and can store up to 1.5 litres of urine until it is able to be voided via the urethra, a small tube which has a sphincter under voluntary control.

Bowel elimination

Just as with other activities of daily living we all have different bowel opening habits. However, usually we open our bowels daily or every other day. Sometimes we may pass loose watery stools: this is called diarrhoea. Other times we may not be able to pass the stool as it may be too hard and painful: this is called constipation. There are many different reasons for these conditions, most of them innocent and with no serious medical implications.

Some people experience frequent changes in bowel habits, for example constipation followed by diarrhoea followed by constipation, etc. This could be a sympton of malignancy in the bowel and should be investigated immediately, but it could also indicate other less severe conditions such as colitis or diverticulitis. Sometimes blood and mucus are passed rectally. The best rule of thumb is to report any change of bowel habits that last longer than a day or two to the doctor.

The patient with bowel problems may lose weight drastically, will often feel lethargic and eventually may become anaemic.

Other factors can cause changes in bowel habit:

- *Drugs* can cause constipation and/or diarrhoea, especially some antibiotics and painkillers.

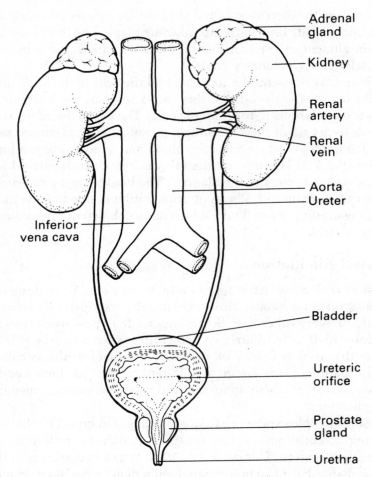

Fig. 7.2 The urinary system. From Jackson S.M. and Bennett P.J. (1988) *Physiology with anatomy for nurses*. London: Baillière Tindall.

- *Immobility,* whether through chronic illness (for example rheumatoid arthritis) or through acute illnesses (for example fractured leg, slipped disc).
- *Change of diet/water,* for example when on holiday or in hospital.
- *Poor diet,* lacking in roughage. Roughage is needed to give faeces bulk so that the muscular action (peristalsis) can act on the faeces.

- *Worry/anxiety*: since the bowel is under the nervous system's control, anxiety of any sort can cause changes in bowel habits.
- *Dehydration*, which may be the result of excessive sweating or heat exhaustion, or an inadequate fluid intake.

Diarrhoea

The commonest cause of diarrhoea is due to the eating of certain types of foods, for example oranges and highly spiced foods. For each individual there may be a particular foodstuff which can cause loose stools. Infections such as gastroenteritis or food poisoning by some other organism, for example salmonella, can be dangerous, especially to the very young and the elderly. Diarrhoea from these infections can lead to dehydration (depletion of body fluids) and this can be very serious. Medical advice should always be sought if the diarrhoea lasts longer than a couple of days or if the patient is not able to take fluids or is vomiting.

When caring for the patient with diarrhoea, medical advice must be sought to eliminate any serious medical condition, but once this has been ruled out good care should keep the patient clean and comfortable. The patient should be nursed in bed and offered clear fluids frequently. In the home it may be helpful to note the amount of fluids the patient is tolerating in case the doctor asks. If in hospital, the amount tolerated should be noted on the fluid balance chart, together with the measured amount of diarrhoea the patient passes.

The anal area of the patient with diarrhoea will probably be very red and sore due to the acidity of the loose stools and therefore care should be taken that it is washed and dried thoroughly. A barrier cream such as zinc and castor oil cream should be applied to protect the delicate skin.

Many patients may be acutely embarrassed about the smell from the diarrhoea so that tact must be used when cleaning away the faeces, especially if bedpans or commodes are used. A small amount of disinfectant diluted with water in the bottom of the commode may help. Always remember the necessity for you and your patient to wash your hands!

Care of the patient with constipation

The patient may be prescribed enemas by the GP and these are given by the district nurse to clear the rectum of the hard faeces. Aperients should only be taken if prescribed by the doctor. A high roughage diet with plenty of fluid is the best method of achieving a regular bowel motion but the patient may have to be taught about which foods are high in roughage. As far as possible one should avoid regular enemata or suppositories.

Make a list of high roughage foods, then turn to the end of this chapter for some examples.

Incontinence

Urinary incontinence

Urinary incontinence, when the urine is voided without any control from the individual, is much more common than faecal incontinence. Control of urination does not develop fully until the child is normally in the second or third year of life and only when the child can control his or her bowel movements. The control depends upon the development of certain parts of the brain and spinal cord, so that people who are brain damaged or have spinal cord damage may be unable to control these body functions and may need help to stay clean and dry. This can be very embarassing for the person and the carer must show tact and consideration at all times. This is especially true where the person once had control and has now lost it, since he or she would have been prepared in childhood to treat these matters in private. Also, however secure any appliance seems, accidents can happen and these create further anxiety and a loss of confidence.

There are three types of urinary incontinence, described below.

Stress incontinence

Stress incontinence is usually found in women who have weakness in their pelvic muscles due to childbirth. The slightest raise in pressure on the bladder, as a result of, for example, sneezing, coughing or laughing, can cause a release of urine. Pelvic floor exercises are now taught to women postnatally to retrain the muscles and establish pelvic muscle control.

Urgency/frequency

Just as children 'when they want to go, have to go' there are occasions when adults experience the same problem. Someone who complains of not being able to hold their urine or who tells you that they are now getting up several times in the night should be advised to mention it to their nurse or doctor. You may have to report this to the nurse in charge since this is often caused by medical conditions, such as cystitis, that are easily treated.

Dribbling

The prostate gland plays an important part in reproduction but, like all glands, secretion slows down with age. In some men this gland becomes hard and causes the neck of the bladder to lose its elasticity, causing pressure, which results in first of all the problems of urgency and frequency, followed by an almost constant dripping. Treatment for this is very routine surgery, so the problem should be mentioned to the doctor or the nurse. Whilst the patient is undergoing investigations or waiting for surgery, there are suitable catheters or condom appliances available that can be used to ensure that he remains dry and comfortable.

It is worth noting that occasionally an enlarged prostate gland may be malignant, so ensure that your patient does seek help, without worrying him too much!

Encouraging continence

Sometimes it is possible to retrain the bladder. This can be achieved by regular toileting. Start off by encouraging the patient to visit the toilet every two hours and extend or reduce the time by 15 minutes until the optimum time has reached the limit. This is by far the management of choice, as the patient feels more independent and, together with the use of well selected aids, can feel confident and maintain his or her self-esteem.

The selection of continence aids can be made easier with the help of a continence adviser. This is a RGN with further training into the problems of incontinence. Most health centres will be able to refer the patient to incontinence clinics attached to local hospitals for help. It is important that you ask the nurse to come and visit any patient who complains of incontinence so that he or she can assess the cause and proceed to plan the patient's care appropriately.

Case histories

Mrs Grundy, aged 82, fell four weeks ago and sprained her knee. She now has difficulty walking quickly or climbing stairs. She complains to you that she increasingly wets herself. Could it be that she is unable to concentrate on two things at once—walking with difficulty and holding her bladder sphincter taut? Would she be helped if you suggested she walked slowly to the toilet every hour rather than waiting until she wanted to go?

John Solomon is 26 and still complains of bed wetting at night following a bad back injury last year. The nurse knows that he had a catheter in his bladder for several months after the accident and that this weakened his sphincter. Although he has no problem in the day, he 'dribbles' at night. A tactful visit from the continence adviser ensures that he has a suitable appliance—and a dry bed!

If the patient is bedridden the aids needed for the patient's comfort may very likely be different from those required by the ambulant (mobile) patient. In some cases the bedridden patient may require a catheter (especially if he/she is unconscious and cannot be placed on a bedpan) or have a urinal kept in place.

However, there may be occasions when catheters are unsuited to the patient or unwanted by the patient and/or relatives. Therefore extra care must be taken to ensure that the patient is never lying on damp sheets (see Chapter 8). There are sheets available commercially and perhaps from local health centres that soak the urine one way and leave the patient lying on a dry area.

Collection of urine/faeces samples

In hospital or in the home, you may be asked to collect a specimen of urine or faeces for investigation.

To collect a sample of faeces

In hospital a papier mâché or ordinary bedpan can be placed on top of the toilet for the patient to use, taking care to ensure that the patient is safe and secure. The patient must be told what is expected and the reason for the collection so that he does not dispose of the sample. Next a small amount of faeces can be placed in the sterile specimen jar (most jars contain a small spatula for this purpose).

In the home this procedure can be difficult if there is no commode and a visit to the local health centre could be useful to get a papier mâché bedpan, which can then be fixed on the toilet. If the patient at home is bedridden then a support for the papier mâché bedpan should also be supplied temporarily from the health centre.

To collect a sample of urine

A urine sample is often called an MSSU (a midstream specimen of urine). This procedure should be carefully and fully explained to the patient. The patient is asked to first pass some urine into the toilet and to stop halfway through. The next stream is passed into a bedpan or bottle and the patient is told to stop halfway through again. Finally, the remaining urine is passed into the toilet. The collected urine is poured carefully into a sterile specimen bottle.

You must always remember to protect yourself when collecting specimens as excreta may be infectious: always wear gloves, avoid splashing and wash your hands thoroughly after any procedure involving excreta.

Testing of urine (urinalysis)

Diabetics are usually required to test their urine for sugar at least
once a day. If you are caring for someone who is a diabetic you
should ask the nurse to show you how to do this correctly.

If you are working in a clinic, particularly a maternity clinic,
you may be required to test the urine of patients attending.
Again, you will need to be shown how to do these tests and
should read the instructions supplied with the test equipment.
On all occasions you must remember to report any findings to
the nurse who is responsible for the patient.

There may be occasions when the smell of a patient's urine tells
you that he or she has a problem. Urine that is infected is cloudy
and smells fishy, whereas an unstable diabetic passes urine that
smells of acetone (nail varnish remover or pear drops). Everyone
is familiar with the colour of normal urine; urine that has blood
in it is much darker in colour (**NB** if there is fresh blood in the
urine, ask the lady if she is menstruating), and there are many
drugs on the market, as well as foods such as beetroot, which
change the colour of urine. In all these instances you must report
your findings to the nurse so that she can investigate the cause.

Colostomy and ileostomy

In some conditions, such as cancer of the bowel or bladder or
ulcerative colitis, the patient may need to have an ileostomy or
colostomy. These are unnatural openings of the colon (in the
case of colostomy) or of the ileum (in the case of ileostomy) and
both open into the stomach wall. They are usually referred to as
stomas.

You are unlikely to be caring for anyone alone who has had an
operation recently and most people, once out of hospital, need
little help unless they are physically handicapped or impaired.
You must be shown how to assist your patient to change their
bags; if you have not done this before, let the nurse know so that
she can teach and then supervise you.

If the bag does not fit correctly leakage will occur and the skin
around the opening will become sore. The patient may also
become embarrassed by the smell. Choosing the correct
appliance and making sure that it fits correctly is a skilled job. If

your patient is having problems you must ask the nurse to visit. Some health authorities employ specialist stoma nurses who have done extra training and it may be that they can advise your patients on new appliances or methods that suit them better.

People with stomas may need to avoid certain foods and some alcoholic drinks; there is no hard and fast rule about this—only trial and error will tell them what they can and cannot eat. Remember that there are supplementary benefits for patients who require special diets; the nurse or social worker will advise on these.

Most urine can safely be passed down the toilet or bedpan washer. The exception to this is if you are working in a hospital caring for a patient with a radioactive implant. If this is the case you must follow the directions and advice of the nurse in charge.

Faeces can be disposed of in the same way. You must make sure that the bedpan is cleaned properly.

Some stoma bags can be emptied into the toilet from the bottom and you will be shown how to do this. Those that do not empty must be dealt with in the same way as soiled dressings and each health authority has its own guidelines for collection of this material. The nurse in charge will explain this to you.

AIDS (acquired immune deficiency syndrome)

There is an increasing number of patients with AIDS being cared for in hospital and at home. The AIDS virus spreads through the blood and body products which contain blood cells. If you are caring for a patient with AIDS there are strict guidelines to be followed to protect yourself and other people. You *must* obtain a copy of these guidelines from the nurse in charge and make sure that she explains these to you. There are also strict controls for the disposal of such things as dressings, catheters and stoma bags.

Conclusion

Ensuring that someone you are caring for is clean and dry and retains as much private control as is possible requires consideration and tact. Learning control or adapting to the lack of it can take time, effort and considerable patience from both of you.

Our knowledge of how to help these people is growing rapidly so do not be afraid to ask the nurse or doctor for advice if the methods you are using do not help the patient as much as you would wish.

We are all aware of how personal and private elimination is. It is even more personal and private for the elderly and for those whose religion directs a different level of morality than we are used to or who have restrictions on who exactly can give care. For example some religions insist that women who are menstruating or who have just had a child are isolated, whilst others have specific rules about handling body washes, diet and sexual behaviour. Remember the health authority guidelines can advise you on appropriate care for your patient.

Foods containing fibre:
- Wholemeal bread
- Nuts
- Fresh fruits
- Fresh vegetables (if not overcooked)
- Baked beans
- Many breakfast cereals (see packets)

8

Meeting hygiene needs

One of the things most people do every day is to wash, shower or bath for the purpose of 'keeping clean', yet this habit has become much more than a purely physical requirement. For both young and old people it is a way of maintaining self-respect and providing relaxation. You must bear this in mind when helping a patient to wash or when attending to other relative hygiene needs.

Skin, hair and nails

Understanding the function of the skin, hair and nails helps us to appreciate why personal hygiene is important.

The main function of the skin is protection. The skin is the largest organ of the body with responsibility for protecting the underlying tissues from injury and infection, assisting in the regulation of body temperature, warning against pain and other external factors such as temperature and pressure (using millions of nerve endings on the skin surface) and prevention of water, protein and salt loss. Dirty skin cannot perform these functions adequately. Overlong nails, dirty nails or torn cuticles can inhibit the protective function of the nails as well as providing a source of infection.

We have hair all over our bodies except for the soles of our feet and the palms of our hands. Like most mammals, hair provides us with one way of regulating our body temperature. When we are cold, small erectile muscles connected to each hair (Fig. 8.1) contract and make the hair stand upright, forming 'goose

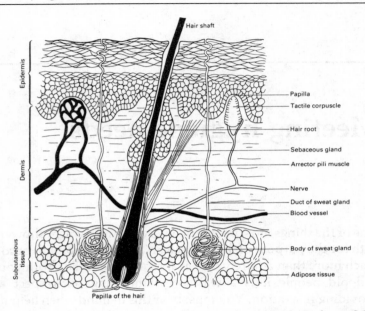

Fig. 8.1   Mammal skin structure seen in section. From Jackson S.M. and Bennett P.J. (1988) *Physiology with anatomy for nurses*. London: Baillière Tindall.

pimples'. These behave like a 'string vest', trapping air between the hairs and acting as insulation by conserving heat within the body. When we are hot the small muscles relax and the hair lies flat against our skin, thus allowing the heat in our body to disperse into the air.

Observe a dog's coat in the winter and again in the summer.

We must remember that hair harbours bacteria and therefore if not kept clean the bacteria can gain entry into the skin and cause spots and pimples.

Each day our skin is producing cells at the basement membrane which travel through the dermis to the epidermis. The epidermis is sometimes known as the 'false skin' as it has no blood supply and is constantly being shed with daily washing and general activities.

Take a slip of sellotape and stick it to the underside of your wrist. Remove it and look at the sellotape. What do you see?

It takes four to five days from production of the skin cell at the basement membrane to the shedding on the surface. When we are ill and unable to wash, a debris of shed skin cells are left on the surface of our skin. These, together with a sticky fluid called sebum secreted from the sebaceous glands, can decompose on the surface of the skin and eventually begin to smell. The true purpose of the sebaceous gland is to produce sebum which keeps the skin supple and waterproof and lubricates the hair. It has a mild antiseptic quality but is greasy and therefore harbours millions of microorganisms.

Sweat glands also lie in the dermis and open into the epidermis at the 'pore'. They produce sweat which consists mainly of water and salts. In hot weather whilst exercising or when 'running a temperature' these glands produce sweat. This is the second method that the skin has of regulating body temperature—as the sweat cools down so the skin also cools.

Minute microorganisms live in harmony on our skin; they only become hazardous when they get through a cut or other injury and gain entry into the delicate underlying tissues. In this warm moist environment they multiply and can cause infection. Similarly, microorganisms from the nose and throat can be passed via our hands to our food and drink, so causing gastric infections if we fail to pay attention to our personal hygiene and that of our patients. The microorganisms can easily be removed from our skin by bathing with soap and water.

Washing, bathing and showering

Although many younger people bath or shower daily we must remember that this may not be the routine for many older people. Remember also that the elderly may find daily bathing detrimental to their skin, causing dryness, and leave them chilled for some time afterwards.

People may have a preference between bathing and showering and if your patient is physically capable of such activities then obviously he or she should have a choice where possible. Apart from the common aids to bathing, such as non-slip mats and handrails, the nurse will know of many more. If money is a problem the DSS can often help.

However, when illness prevents normal bathing you will have to assist with bed bathing. Where possible it is pleasant to have a bed bath at the same time of day that one would normally bath. However, hospital routine may not allow this.

Bed bathing

The room should be warm and free from draughts. The curtains of a hospital cubicle must be drawn, allowing the patient to feel private. During this procedure the patient should never be exposed unduly. The patient should dictate the speed of the bed bath and you must remember that bed bathing can be tiring if attacked too vigorously.

The necessary equipment must be gathered together, including bowl, hot and cold water, flannels, combs, soap, towels and any other toiletries to avoid leaving the patient alone during the bed bath. You must allow the patient to feel the water to see if it is the correct temperature. Allow the patient to wash and dry himself as much as possible without overtiring himself. This gives a sense of achievement and allows the patient to feel dignified. Also it is easier for himself to dry himself than for you to do this.

Attention should be given to the eyelids, always washing away from the centre but remember that eyes are self-cleansing, so there is no need for vigorous washing.

There is no particular order in which to wash the body and the best method is the one that suits your relative or patient, remembering only that the area in between the legs (the genitalia) and the bottom are the last to be washed, preferably with a separate, disposable cloth.

Hair care in bed

As already stated, the skin is constantly being shed and this applies also to the skin on top of the head. This may cause irritation to the patient. You may be required to wash the hair of a bedridden patient; ask the nurse to demonstrate how to do this quickly and comfortably.

The hair should be dried, with a hair dryer if required, into the style that the patient desires. This procedure can be exhausting and it may be important to allow the patient to rest afterwards.

Cultural considerations

Remember that Britain has become a multicultural society and it would be impossible, either in a hospital or in the community, for you to avoid becoming involved with the care of people from varying cultural backgrounds. You must therefore be aware of any special requirements when attending to these people's hygiene. A few important differences are considered below.

Hinduism

Hindus must perform ceremonial washing several times a day. They have symbols on their bodies that must never be removed, for example a married woman wears a mark in the centre of her forehead near the hairline and men wear a thread around their neck or wrist. The removal of sacred adornments requires a special ceremony. Females may not wish to be cared for by members of the opposite sex.

Islam

Muslims also have ritual washing ceremonies several times a day. They use their right hands for clean tasks and their left hands for unclean tasks. Again, females may not wish to be attended to by male carers.

Sikhism

Male Sikhs will not wish to be shaved as this is not part of their culture. They wear a bangle on their wrist that should never be removed, neither should their sword or comb. Female and male Sikhs wear shorts that must never be completely removed— when bathing or changing clothes one leg only is taken out at any one time.

You must remember and respect different cultural norms and customs—they date back many hundreds of years. Try to adapt your methods of caring to suit the individual. For example many Asians who are ill are reluctant to bath, believing that it can cause further illness and even death. However, they may wipe their skin with cleaning oils or special talcum powder, both of which are effective aids to hygiene care.

Infestation

You are probably aware that infestation of head lice is quite common amongst children due to the close community they find at school. Head lice can be spread rapidly in these sorts of situations. However, adults can get lice too. In a hospital or other type of institution body and head lice can be a real problem. Your first priority is to alert a trained nurse and *calmly* attempt to keep the person isolated from others. You must also protect yourself when attending to the patient. A gown and a scarf is sufficient for this.

The signs that a person is infested are obvious. The person will be itching on either the head or the warm areas on the body, for example under the arms or in between the legs. On further inspection of the head, the nits (eggs) of the lice will be seen attached to the hair close to the scalp. They are yellow in colour and the size of a pinhead. The mature lice can be seen by the eye and are either grey (head lice) or brown (pubic lice).

There are many commercial products that you can buy from the chemist and if in any doubt as to the product to buy the pharmacist will be able to advise. Alternatively, you could seek advice from the district nurse at your local health centre or your local chemist. The instructions for treatment are very easy nowadays and involve simple shampooing with special solutions. A fine tooth comb is usually included in the packs or you can purchase these at your chemist. Finally, it is important that you do not allow your patient to witness disgust or displeasure on your face. He or she may be feeling embarrassed already, and it is your responsibility to reassure, whilst at the same time educating your patient as to the treatment and prevention of further infestation.

Nail care

Nail care is important for hygiene, comfort and self-esteem, for both men and women. You should ask the patients what care they require for their hands and nails. Nails should be cut slightly curved and filed into shape smoothly with an emery board. Nail varnish can be applied if the patient would like and finally moisturising cream can be rubbed into the hands and nails to prevent chafing and to keep the hands supple. A hand massage can be very relaxing.

Foot care

Toe nails should be attended to as frequently as finger nails. Often the elderly are unable to reach their feet and they can become neglected. This can lead to immobility in many cases, as the nails can become ingrown or the nail of the great toe can become thickened and horny. This is known as a Ram's horn toe nail. Normally the toe nails should be cut straight across to prevent ingrowth, but in cases like Ram's horn or simple thickening it is necessary to contact the chiropodist. In the community, chiropodists hold clinics in the local health centre. However, if your patient or relative is unable to get to the centre, chiropodists can make domiciliary visits if referred by the GP or other members of the health centre team in the health centre.

NB Patients who are diabetic may have circulatory problems and you must *never* attempt to cut difficult toe nails of these patients—instead refer them to a trained nurse. Do not allow relatives, or the patient, to cut toe nails in such cases. Severe infection may result if the nails are badly cut or the skin is damaged.

Conclusion

Even when we are ill it remains important to feel dignified and maintain our self-esteem; in fact, it is perhaps much more important at these times. In more recent years greater emphasis has been placed upon the patient's feelings of self-worth. You will always have to consider in which ways you can enable your patient to feel better psychologically. Being shaved, having hair styled or set, make-up applied, moustache trimmed, nail varnish applied, or even a hand or foot massage can aid the patient to feel much brighter.

Nowadays young and old alike have become aware of the importance of appearance, so do not assume that the older the patient is the less concerned they are regarding their appearance.

9

Waking and dressing

As with all daily routines we each have our own way of doing things and our own preferences. Waking up in the morning and getting dressed are no exceptions. You will be involved with helping people to get up and it is important that you find out the patient's own routine and likes and dislikes; as far as possible try to adhere to them. For instance, some people may like to have a drink prior to rising; others, however, may need to go to the toilet immediately; you must adapt your care to the needs of the patient.

Ask different members of your family and friends what *they* do immediately on waking. Make a list of their different routines.

By continuing with the patient's own routine you will help him feel more secure and make the process of being helped and dependent on others less stressful. Remember that your aim is to help someone rise and dress in a safe and dignified manner.

One of the first things you should do prior to getting someone out of bed and dressed is to look around the room or area you are to work in and ask yourself several questions.

- Is the room warm enough for the patient? First you need to ask the patient how he or she feels. Then touch the patient's arms and legs—how do they feel? Warm or cold to the touch? If the room is not warm enough or the patient feels cool, then check that all the windows and doors are closed and then try to heat the room with electric, solid fuel or gas fires. If this is not possible you will have to use blankets to cover the patient. If they are not available, or if the patient feels cold all over, or if the weather is very cold you will have to decide to leave the patient in bed and inform your manager. (This applies especially in winter with elderly or frail patients who might be at risk of hypothermia.) (See Chapters 4 and 9.)

- Is there plenty of space for me to work in? If not, remove bits of furniture or equipment to allow yourself and the patient room to move. However, you must always ask permission if you are in the patient's own home and replace the furniture afterwards.

- Is the equipment I might need all here (for example clothes, blankets, hair brush, bowl, soap, etc)? If not, collect all the equipment you need before you begin and explain what you are doing to the patient.

- Have all the hazards been removed, such as small rugs and carpets, dogs, cats, etc? If not and you are in the patient's own home, ask if you might remove them for a short while and explain the reasons, for example if the patient is unsteady when standing or if there is insufficient room for you to work safely.

Before the patient gets out of bed offer the patient a drink. This not only allows the patient time to wake properly but also gives you the time to prepare the room and collect the bits and pieces you need. It may also be necessary for the patient to take analgesics (painkillers) prior to moving to stop pain in joints, bones, etc. This is common with conditions such as rheumatoid arthritis, osteoarthritis and muscular strains.

NB Remember that some people may have taken sleeping tablets and can be unsteady on their feet. *Find out if they have.*

Before a patient is dressed he or she may need a bed bath or a chair bath as opposed to just washing hands and face. However, with dressing you still have to bear in mind the same principles of privacy as with bathing. The patient should *never* be exposed unnecessarily; consider how you would feel sitting naked in front of an acquaintance.

After you have washed or bathed your patient, hearing aids, glasses and dentures should be cleaned and replaced, as these are important aids for the patient to communicate. You should check that all these aids are in good working order and that they fit correctly. Badly fitting aids can cause redness and tenderness of the skin tissue around them, for example around the ears, nose and in the mouth. If you do notice any redness or tenderness report to your manager promptly.

Whilst you are helping with personal hygiene and dressing, the patient may feel embarrassment and awkwardness; chatting can often be a useful sociable distraction but you will have to know if this is what your patient likes to do first thing in the morning. Some people might prefer to listen to the radio, watch the television or simply be quiet whilst getting up and dressed.

At some point whilst getting someone up it may be necessary to transfer them from bed to chair or toilet. The process of moving and lifting people is covered in Chapter 4 but it is important at this stage to warn against attempting to move or lift without adequate training. If you feel you cannot move or lift a patient then do not attempt to but ask your manager about training.

NB Remember that your responsibility is to your own health as well as to your patient's.

It may be that the problems you and your patient are having with 'transferring' is due to some simple factor, for example the bed may be too high. With permission this can easily be solved by cutting down the wooden legs. The bed may also be too low, in which case bed blocks can be made or the DSS may be able to put you in touch with a place to hire such blocks. The same department may be able to help in getting a divan bed for the patient.

Dressing

The way we dress reflects our personality: for example when we feel happy and confident we may choose to wear bold clothes; at other times we may feel quite introverted and shy and then we may choose subtle clothes. Unfortunately, in many hospitals this is not borne in mind and the patients may find themselves in clothes that they would never choose for themselves. Whether you are working in the patient's home or hospital you should let the patient choose what he would like to wear.

There are certain physical disabilities that limit the selection of certain clothes but with some thought a solution to these problems can be found. For example, if the patient has to have quick access to the toilet to pass urine or empty his bowels, instead of leaving underwear off, which is the present practice in many hospitals, properly fitted back opening underpants or crutchless knickers can be the acceptable answer and make the condition less stressful and more manageable for the patient.

When selecting materials to make clothes for patients you can give good advice about certain fabrics to be considered. It is always good policy to have inflammable nightwear, especially with children and the frail elderly patient. There may also be a need for water resistant material if the patient is incontinent or prone to spilling drink or food. You can also advise about fabric protector spray which can easily be applied to certain materials making them waterproof. Drip dry material prevents the need for ironing—ideal for arthritic patients—and well fitting, comfortable shoes are essential.

Once the patient has chosen his or her clothes you should help where necessary to dress but it is important to remember to let the patient do as much as possible for him/herself without pain. You have to ensure that the clothing is suitable (not too warm in summer, not too cool in winter) and that you leave a blanket or cardigan within reach. Anyone who needs help dressing obviously has some immobility problem and will not be able to keep warm by moving about the house. The old also tend to feel the cold.

Shoes can be a problem for many incapacitated people as they are difficult to tie and also one has to bend down to fit them on. Long shoe horns prevent this bending and elasticated shoe laces and slip-on shoes make this procedure easier.

Helping to dress someone does not finish at clothing. Hair is another important part of dressing. You will need to be guided by the patient or his relatives as to what style he likes and is used to. Perfume or aftershave should be applied if required and do not forget jewellery and watches; these are important finishing touches. A mirror should be available to enable the patients to check on the way they look.

Finally, patients should be left comfortable with all the necessary personal items around them.

Make a list of items that a patient may need nearby, for example books, magazines, writing materials, etc.

Remember that many patients at home have caring relatives who wish to help them. You will be in the position to enable them to do this and with tact you can teach your skills to them. By helping their relatives they will feel useful and perhaps less frustrated.

Getting someone up and dressed correctly can set the scene for the day. If carried out properly it can be pleasurable for the patient and yourself. It should never be a rushed activity and you should consider carefully how to make it less stressful for the patient.

Cultural considerations

Remember that people from differing cultures will wear the dress to which they are accustomed and in which they feel comfortable. Cultural identity is important for all and clothing helps to maintain this. You may require help from the family to understand the dress.

There are various health authority booklets to help you understand the various modes of dress that you may experience. Ask your manager if there is such a booklet in your area.

Financial support

In some emergency situations such as theft or fire or if a person has lost or gained weight rapidly, an interest-free crisis loan may be obtained from the Social Fund of the DSS. The method is to apply through social security offices and an example of claims paid for certain articles can be found at the local Citizens Advice Bureau (CAB).

The Salvation Army run a family service centre and have two

Table 9.1 Aids to waking and dressing

Waking	Dressing	
	Clothes	Equipment
Rope ladder (to pull upright in bed)	Slash-back dresses, shirts, nightwear	Long handled shoehorns
Bed blocks	Elastic waist bands	Dressing sticks
	Trousers with drop front pouch/front fastenings	Stocking pullers
	Velcro fastenings	
	Elastic laces	

systems for distribution of clothing. Nationally they run clothing shops where people can get articles of clothing for next to nothing. They also have facilities for giving clothes away free in special circumstances, for example fire, unemployment, etc. To obtain more information, the Salvation Army will help. You will find their number in the local telephone directory.

Oxfam and the WRVS also run clothing shops that you can contact.

Aids to waking and dressing are summarised in Table 9.1. The Disabled Living Foundation give advice for adapting clothing.

10

Encouraging independence

The activities of living we have so far discussed have related more to the physical aspects of health—safety and cleanliness and so on. As human beings, however, we need much more than that. To have a sense of worth and achievement is important to us. We possess the most complex brains in the animal kingdom and these need nourishing and satisfying in just the same way as the rest of our bodies. The food they need, however, is rather more abstract: an opportunity to be active, to achieve our goals in life at work and play, to be stimulated by new challenges, interests and a sense of learning. We like to feel in control of our lives and our health, even when we rely upon others for help, so that we can exercise choice in the course of our lives. Helping patients in these respects is just as important as bathing somebody correctly or making sure they have the correct diet.

Imagine that you are ill and confined to bed or unable to be independent because of paralysis or severe arthritis. What sort of things would be important to you to keep you interested and happy with life?

Boredom can be as lethal as any illness. It makes us feel dull and uninteresting—to ourselves and to others. We may feel helpless, less human or an object to which other people do things beyond our control. We become unhappy, worry about ourselves and our problems and forget the wider world. We may experience feelings of worthlessness, becoming depressed and perhaps even suicidal.

Coping with a health problem or disability can be an immense task for any patient. Add to it the feelings described above and the sense of loss, inadequacy and hopelessness can become overwhelming.

It is not enough to keep someone occupied on some pointless task or just to 'jolly them along'. It is no use giving someone something to do simply to pass the time; for example basket weaving is of little value unless the patient is actually interested in basket weaving. Time which is passed is time which is lost.

In hospitals and communities certain professionals are employed (occupational therapists) who specialise in the management of these difficulties and you should consult an expert of this type if possible to help your patient with problems of boredom and frustration. They are also expert at teaching patients how to help themselves, for example how to dress and wash again after a stroke. To be able to 'do' for ourselves is an important contribution to our sense of well-being and achievement.

However, before approaching the occupational therapist, there are many simple strategies you can follow to help people in your day to day contacts with them. Here are a few suggestions:

- Find out whether there is a local day centre or rehabilitation unit available where the patient can go for occupational therapy and expert help towards independence and relief of boredom.
- Adopt a style of nursing that makes the patient feel that he or she is 'in charge' of his or her own body and mind. Your role is that of helper, teacher and adviser, not that of a god controlling the patient's destiny and denying all choice in his or her care.
- Make your patient feel important. Listen to his feelings and try to help him solve his problems, referring to the relevant professionals where appropriate.
- Encourage visitors and others to maintain their contacts with the patient and help you in your plan of activities.
- Use praise and positive words of encouragement at every

opportunity. It is better to say 'well done, John, you've eaten almost all your soup yourself today' than 'what a mess, you've spilled some again'.

- Find out what your patient's interests are. Get to know him, his history, his family, his job, his hobbies. Show an interest in what they are.
- Find common areas of interest that you can talk about honestly and sincerely.
- Try to provide the things the patient needs to maintain hobbies and interests as much as possible, for example books, modelling equipment, stamp collections, radio, TV (especially if his favourite programme is on). Try to 'fill in' by helping with those things which he cannot do himself: read for the blind patient, help the disabled swimmer to get to the baths, take your patient shopping, to the theatre, the cinema, the football match or just for a walk outdoors (check first with a trained nurse or with the hospital).
- Find suitable sources of recreation that your patient can manage. A patient who is very ill may have little concentration. A magazine may be better to read than a book. A short TV programme is preferable to a long film. Shopping by post may be an alternative to a shopping trip. Large print books are better for the visually handicapped, while talking books (tape recordings) can replace the written text.
- Show the patient that you care for him and accept him as he is. Spend time with him, listen to him (rather than talk to him). Be sincerely friendly and affectionate. A friendly cuddle or holding someone's hand speaks volumes to someone who is lonely and unhappy. Touch between people is a vital part of communication; it makes us feel welcome, loved and accepted. Remember that many people feel lonely and unloved because they are rarely touched, for example an elderly patient without relatives, a widow who lives alone, a child who is severely physically handicapped.
- When working towards choice and independence do not set your target too far ahead. Expecting too much of your patient may lead him to give up in despair. A few steps achieved successfully and gradually increased at the bedside is far more rewarding than expecting him to walk the full length of the

room. Choose activities that the patient can manage or suggest new ones, for example swimming when football is no longer available.

- Join with them in group games and activities. Laugh and have fun with them. Use reminiscence or items of common interest to strike up conversation, for instance introduce a patient who has lived in the same area or worked at the same job, or who shares similar hobbies. Have items about the ward or room which are of interest to your patient—personal things or things which become a source of interest or conversation. For example a picture of a Lancaster Bomber in a hospital ward will spark off many conversations and reminiscences among the elderly patients about wartime days. Photographs of babies serve the same purpose on a maternity ward.
- Apart from inanimate objects (a picture, a favourite piece of furniture) there are also the animate to consider. When in hospital, is it not possible for the ward to have a pet cat, fish or budgie for the patients? Could the patient's much loved pet not be brought in to visit him?
- Remember not to spend most time with the patients you particularly like or who are the easy jokers or conversationalists. The quiet patients or those with problems of sight, speech or hearing need your help and company just as much as others.
- Find out what other sources of help are available—social clubs, Meals on Wheels, home helps, church groups, etc. There are also many societies which offer support and social activities for people with specific difficulties (for example Parkinson's Disease Society)—see the list of these on page 178.
- Find out what possible aids can help your patient to be more independent—from wheelchairs to walking frames, modified typewriters to talking books. Trained staff will be able to advise you on the many appropriate aids available. The Possum (patient operated selector system) is a kind of type-writer which allows disabled people to select a number of different functions, including typing and operating the equipment.
- Compare and contrast your own lifestyle with that of the person you are caring for. How often do they see people? How

often do they 'get out'? Although we often complain our own life is 'too busy' or 'too tiring' it takes very little imagination to realise how dull and lonely the lives are of those who need care.

- Investigate the possibility of holidays. Many groups or societies can offer expert advice on holidays for the disabled and most reputable hotels, travel agents, airlines, etc, will offer valuable guidance on what they can do to help.
- Many *further education* opportunities are available either at home or in colleges or schools. Almost every local college has special courses for the less able and special interest or hobbies courses. There are also pre and post-retirement courses, Open University courses, etc. Increasing disability may rule out old pleasures but new skills and hobbies can be developed as replacements. It is not true that 'you can't teach an old dog new tricks'.
- Become aware of the difficulties and frustrations of the less able yourself. Persuade someone to push you around your local town in a wheelchair. It is a salutary experience! Many public places may be quite inaccessible to you and there is the frustration of people talking down to you. Perhaps you might participate more in your local community by asking shop-keepers and local councils to provide more and better access for the disabled.
- Attend to your patient's environment (see Chapter 3 for more details) with flowers, pictures, clean and comfortable furniture and access to a garden or a window with an open view.
- Provide information on the management of the patient's health problems. Take his views into account and participate in teaching him how to manage his treatment. He can be provided with sources of contact for help and advice. Be ready to refer the patient to a doctor or nurse for expert advice when appropriate. If the patient is very disabled you may have to take over many of these responsibilities completely, such as giving him his medicines on time and making sure he gets his regular check-ups at the GP or dentist.

There are an enormous range of possibilities for you to think about and act upon. Providing interest, recreation and exercise is a vital part of the helping relationship with your patient. Perhaps you have realised that there is no such thing as 'nothing can be done' to help relieve serious boredom or unhappiness. For every patient, there is always something. Consider which social activities you participate in that could be opened to the disabled if only someone would transport them to and from home!

Most of the illnesses that we and our patients will suffer from are known as *acute illnesses*. The illness can start suddenly, is treated either medically or surgically and then, over a period of time, the patient should recover and return to his or her normal lifestyle and routines. 'Flu, appendicitis and gallstones are examples of acute illnesses.

A *chronic illness* develops and is, at the present time, incurable, although if this condition is treated correctly, is not life threatening. These illnesses (for example cerebral vascular accident, arthritis, multiple sclerosis and diabetes) can prevent us from resuming the same lifestyle that we are used to without some adaptation either physically, socially, sexually or mentally. When these and other chronic illnesses happen, we have to deliver our care in a specialised way for our patients, helping them to come to terms with their condition. Perhaps the most important aim is to *care for the patient without depriving him of independence, choice and freedom*. These patients are not children but adults who through disease are unable to care for themselves as well as they would wish to. Coming to terms with this different approach to their lifestyle will probably be the worse problem that the person has to face and it may take time. The patient could be very bitter and appear impatient and ungrateful. You have to understand this and show tact and patience, allowing the patient to exhibit anger and frustration. Eventually most people with chronic illnesses come to terms with what they can and cannot do. The speed of this realisation will depend on your patience, skills and support.

Examples of some chronic diseases

Cerebral vascular accident (stroke)

Cerebral vascular accident (CVA) is the result of an obstruction or rupture of a blood vessel in the brain. The brain cells die due to oxygen deprivation from lack of blood and unfortunately these cells are the only cells in the body that never rejuvenate. The effects of this condition can range from a slight weakness down one side of the body to complete paralysis of one side (for example arm, leg, neck and trunk muscles), which is known as *hemiplegia*.

Sometimes sight, speech and hearing are also affected and as a result the patient has difficulty in understanding and is often labelled 'confused'. Stroke is an extremely complex condition. It may be helpful to ask your district nursing sister or ward sister to explain some of the problems the patient may suffer from or complain of. You could also write to the Chest, Heart and Stroke Foundation (address on page 179). These organisations can give advice and details of support groups as well as producing booklets which will help you to understand the complex nature of this condition.

Osteoarthritis

Osteoarthritis (inflammation of joints) can affect the spine, the hips, knees, ankles and feet. There is no known cause for this condition but obesity does aggravate the symptoms. The individual suffers from pain, stiffness and swelling of the affected joints leading to immobility and, if the hands are affected, difficulty in many activities of daily life, including personal hygiene.

Write down some other activities of daily living which might be difficult for someone with osteoarthritis.

Osteoarthritis is very common in the elderly, so much so that persons might not seek help, just putting their symptoms down to old age, but in fact treatment is quite successful and can give great relief.

In the preceding chapters we have looked at certain aids which can help the individual with activities of daily life. Your local social services department should have a rehabilitation officer who will visit the patient, assess his or her needs and supplies the aids and adaptations needed. There may be a small charge for some items. However, the Disabled Living

Foundation, a voluntary organisation (address on page 179), does have information on aids and adaptations for loan or hire in any area. You may also find the DHSS leaflet HB 2/Nov 80 'Aids for the Disabled' useful; you can get this from local DSS offices or post offices.

Diabetes mellitus

Diabetes is a chronic illness which affects the patient in many ways. The pancreas produces and secretes insulin. Diabetes is a reduction of the insulin from the pancreas. Insulin is necessary for the breakdown of carbohydrates; without it we can become seriously ill and ultimately die. It is therefore necessary for the person to receive treatment. Usually this is for life. The treatment may involve regular tablets and diet or it may involve daily injections of insulin together with a stricter diet. Both treatments mean a drastic change to the patient's regular habits as well as additional routines of medication.

Some diabetics are teenagers who find the new regimen difficult to adopt and may exhibit anger and resentment that this should happen to them at a time of so much change and development. Other diabetic patients are very elderly and although prepared to comply with tablet taking, diet, etc, they may find their new regimen hard to follow, or they may forget and get confused about when to take tablets and diet. You will be guided as to the help that is required of you (urine testing, etc) but perhaps one of the most important things you can do is to be alert to and recognise the early warning symptoms if some thing seems to be going wrong and report it immediately to the nurse in charge, for example if the patient is feeling ill or if you notice certain unpermitted items of food in the house.

Ask your nursing sister to tell you what is involved in a diabetic diet.

Very often the dietician can help the patient and his relatives to understand diet, but adequate preparation should be made to educate those involved prior to the patient being discharged home. It is within your remit to make these procedures as unembarrassing as possible. With suitable aids, a little forethought and some honest discussion between you and your patient, you can help this to be less traumatic.

Coping with loss of mobility resulting from chronic illness

The inability to move when and where we like can have a profound effect on the individual producing frustration, anger and also fear.

Why fear? Close your eyes now, imagine you are stuck where you are now, unable to move out of that place. Now imagine hearing a strange noise, smelling something burning, feeling faint or actually falling off the chair; you are unable to do anything. A feeling of total helplessness is the common reaction.

There was possibly only one other time when we were totally helpless and that was when we were babes in arms. As babies we had little choice where we were put; you must *never* allow the patient to feel that his or her choice has gone. Allow the patient to have control; for example allow him to choose where he would like to sit.

As already stated the client with chronic illness or disability will require long-term help. It is very important therefore to be honest with the client. Honesty is important both for the client's sake, for the relatives' sake and for your own. It is no good pretending that everything will soon get back to normal if it might very well not and the sooner the person faces the anger and frustration of restructuring his or her life, the quicker he or she will be able to enjoy living it.

One of the ways in which we might find enjoyment are with *hobbies and other leisure activities*. These are important not only for relaxation but sometimes for feelings of achievement and satisfaction which we all need at some time. Perhaps previous hobbies will be unsuitable for the patients as they become ill but with adequate searching a new hobby may be found which would once again give these feelings of creativity.

Many chronically disabled people find much enjoyment working for their voluntary organisations for the specific conditions from which they are suffering. Your local CAB can help you find your local group and if there is not one, perhaps you or your client may be interested in starting one.

For many chronically sick or disabled people and their children or partners, formal occupations may not be possible and non-contributory benefits may be obtained from the DSS. The local services will be able to help in this direction by providing leaflets and advice. They will make home visits if needed to advise housebound or very elderly people.

These issues can be broadly described as '*Health education*' and are an important aspect of the modern approach to care. The main aim of health education is prevention of ill health, but there is another aspect, often overlooked, and that is helping individuals to deal with their illness and return to a lifestyle which is as normal as possible. You will be involved with this. The usual good diet, exercise, leisure, good personal hygiene and work of some kind will help maintain and perhaps increase general health of the chronically sick, but you must seek advice to find out what is suggested for your particular client.

Remember that health education means giving the facts, the pros and cons without inflicting guilt and then allowing the individual to make his own choice.

If the patient wants to make changes to his or her lifestyle *then* you can help. Consider the following two examples.

Mr Anderson, a 58 year old man, has recovered from the acute symptoms of a CVA, leaving him with a right hemiplegia (right-sided paralysis). Mr Anderson lives with his wife and mother in a three bedroomed house; recovered well in hospital and was released after six weeks rehabilitation; he can walk with a stick, but cannot yet climb stairs. There is a downstairs toilet with washing facilities. His immediate problems are the need for somewhere to sleep and the fact that he is complaining of constipation.

The first problem is solved by moving his single bed downstairs. However, although an enema solves his immediate problem, health education is needed for a long-term solution. What dietary advice should be offered? And who else may be needed to make a home visit to check that he can eat a healthy diet without discomfort?

Janet Walters a 28 year old typist with ICI, has early stage multiple sclerosis. She is anxious about what to tell her fiancé, what to tell her employers, how she is going to cope and what the future holds.

Janet can be referred to the superb occupational health service at ICI who will arrange her necessary regular injections and may be able to assist her with the counselling she needs as she and her boyfriend come to terms with the future. The occupational health services are also important in assisting her to continue in employment.

In addition, both you and your supervising nurse can offer health education and advice in relation to diet, housing, family planning advice and hobbies. Finally, you can provide someone to talk to by listening yourself and by giving her the address of the local multiple sclerosis support group who will provide more long-term support.

The plan will be prepared by the nurse in charge. It will always be possible to give the patient a feeling of competence and satisfaction. At first when the patient is asked what plans he or she has for the future, they may be unrealistic. If the patient fails to attain such goals, this in itself reinforces failure, so you must be very supportive to ensure that expectations are realistic.

Note for carers of the chronically ill

Caring for these patients is a long-term task: so, even if the patient is a relative, you must always think about your own general health as well as theirs; if you do not, you may eventually need care yourself.

Remember that lifting is a skill with specific principles which must be adhered to. Constant stress on fragile spinal muscles due to bad lifting practices will eventually lead to serious problems causing inconvenience to your relative or client, but a bad back could make you chronically sick, ruining not only your career prospects, but also your personal life. So remember to make sure that you are taught the principles of proper lifting, and if in doubt, ask for refresher courses.

If you are caring for a relative or friend you will need to be aware that you have to have some time off. You will need time to enjoy yourself; we all have to have time for relaxation and leisure to 'replenish our batteries'. Hobbies are an excellent method of relieving tension and therefore are important to you as well. Ask the sister about any support groups which you can join, and do not forget the value of friends. Church members and colleagues are often happy to listen and help where they can. Sometimes it is possible to arrange 'respite care'—short-term admission in hospital whilst carers have a holiday or break.

Always remember that although your skills are important you have limitations. Your aim is to aid the patient as much as possible and this means seeking help where available. Many of the problems that the chronically sick and disabled suffer from or complain of are wrongly attributed to their illness. Never allow a problem to continue without referring it to your nursing sister for assessment. She or the doctor will investigate and most probably be able to alleviate it to some degree.

11

Sexualising

This chapter is not simply about sex—or at least sex in the sense of physical stimulation of the self or others for the purpose of pleasure or procreation. The notion of sexuality goes beyond the stimulation of the sexual organs and enters the realms of the way we think about ourselves and others, and the kind of behaviour that occurs as a result.

As a helper, much that you do directly affects your sexuality and that of the person you are helping. In the helping relationship, you may cross barriers of intimate physical and psychological contact which you would never dream of crossing in your daily life.

Development and changes in our sexuality may occur throughout our lives.

Write down, in two columns headed 'Male' and 'Female', what you think are some of the main sexual 'milestones' in people's lives.

For both men and women you may have noted growing awareness of their own bodies, masturbation, puberty, changes in the sex organs, developing interest in the opposite or same sex, parenthood. The end of women's reproductive capacity comes with menopause, while men may remain fertile into very old age.

You may have noticed already how we tend to talk of a person's 'sex' (i.e. male or female) but think of their sexuality (i.e. the way it is expressed) quite differently from their ability to reproduce. In conversation, we often use the terms inter-changeably. It is not the purpose of this book to be a sex guide for carers; rather we are looking at how we need to take account of the sexuality of both the carer and the cared for—this affects the type of help we give. At this stage, however, it might be a good idea if you made a check of your understanding of the following terms with a good dictionary, before we proceed further.

- Puberty
- Ovum
- Sperm
- Ovaries
- Testes
- Fallopian tubes
- Vas deferens
- Uterus
- Vagina
- Penis
- Mammary glands
- Coitus
- Sexual intercourse
- Masturbation
- Heterosexuality
- Bisexuality
- Homosexuality
- Celibacy
- Lesbianism
- Menopause
- Sterility
- Infertility
- Impotence
- Frigidity

If you have looked at this list in detail, you will see that there is a difference between defining someone's sex (for example they have the sexual characteristics of a man or woman) and defining their sexuality (for example the way they express their sex). Thus we move beyond mere definition of people in terms of their physical attributes (sex, i.e. men have more body hair and a penis; women have breasts and a vagina) into those areas in which they behave with those sexual attributes (sexuality).

This may sound quite simple until we start to think of the implications of these behaviours, especially when they do not fit easily into our view of what is 'normal'. Talking about 'normal' can be very tricky, for the idea of normality tends to shift about a lot according to the society we live in, our individual attitudes and the changes that occur over time.

If you think of normal sexuality as men performing sexual acts exclusively with women, then that narrows down your definition of normal to exclude masturbation or homosexuality. Masturbation was regarded as unhealthy and a sin in Victorian times; now we tend to look upon it as quite a normal thing to do. Homosexuality has been treated with acceptance in some cultures and hostility and repression in others. So, where does that leave us, or more precisely, you?

It is not the purpose of this text to argue the rights and wrongs of different kinds of sexuality. You will have your own views which you have developed over the years. However, as someone involved in helping others you carry some obligations:

- You need to understand how your body and that of the opposite sex works.
- You need to know about the many different ways in which people express their sexuality.
- You must be able to help someone with equal sensitivity, regardless of their sex or sexuality, and to give that help without losing their respect.

If you cannot accept another person without expressing disapproval or making moral judgment about the rights and wrongs of his or her behaviour, then you may come across many instances where you will be unable to help your patient.

Think about how you might respond to the following circumstances:

- A young girl (unmarried) is admitted to hospital for an abortion.
- An elderly man masturbates in front of you.
- A young woman admitted through casualty turns out to be a man in woman's clothing (a transvestite).

- A patient of the opposite or same sex makes a pass at you.
- A friend seeks advice on methods of birth control.

You can see that the circumstances in which we help people can be loaded with our own values and opinions, which might make it very difficult for us to be objective and give equal help in all circumstances.

However, helping with sexuality is not always so complex. A little thought and consideration enables us to do much to support someone's sense of sexuality:

- Helping an elderly lady to choose attractive clothing which she prefers
- Encouraging a young man to select a pleasant after-shave
- Helping with making the hair attractive, applying make-up, shaving, washing, dressing, etc
- Using praise and other words of encouragement (sincerely) to suggest that someone looks good
- Use of touch (holding hands, cuddling) to make someone feel accepted, attractive and loved.

An important role for the helper can be not only to accept someone's sexuality without showing embarrassment, but to help them feel 'normal' (for them) and meet the ways in which they normally express their sexuality, for example in the way they look. The link between the way we look and our sexuality is also important. It affects our sense of being a person, our dignity, our feelings of being man or woman, our feelings of being valued and loved.

Think about the following examples. Apart from the matter of the healing of their injuries, what feelings might the patients have in these circumstances, about the way they look, how attractive they are to others, or how far they might still feel fully a man or a woman?

- A young man with severe facial scarring after a motor cycle accident
- A young woman who has had a breast removed because of cancer

- An elderly lady with facial and body paralysis on one side of her body
- A middle-aged man who has had an operation which has not only made him infertile and impotent, but also requires regular dressings in his genital area

Many of the complex issues discussed above are involved here. Perhaps you can see that diseases, injuries or operations which affect our appearance, our sexual organs, or our ability to take care of our own appearance can also have implications for the way we view our 'body image' and our sexuality.

Given the above difficulties, how can you help? Perhaps you could try discussing the above examples with colleagues and friends, to identify the sort of help that *you* might prefer in the difficult circumstances mentioned. The following major points need to be considered:

- You must gain a knowledge of the human body and how it works, particularly in relation to those organs primarily concerned with sexuality.
- Patients need your acceptance and understanding of their difficulties: no looks of horror when you see the injured face; no forgetting that the woman can be just as worried about her appearance and sexuality as the healing of her breast wound.
- Refer to expert counsellors and senior nurses and medical staff for advice and guidance in giving your patients care.
- Privacy is important when dealing with intimate procedures, dressings, bathing, toiletting, etc, as is time to be alone and in private with relatives and loved ones. For example, could an elderly couple in long-stay care, be offered the same room to share or perhaps the same bed?
- Confidentiality must be assured. Very personal things about the patients should be known only to the caring staff.
- Help patients to deal with the problems themselves, with words of praise to encourage them when they do well; for example teach the older lady to apply her make-up and attend to her hair as she normally would.
- Help other people whom the patients may contact to accept and understand their difficulties. For example introduce

patients with similar problems or explain to other patients what to expect, in order to remove the 'shock' element. Again, you will need to refer to a senior nurse about this.

- Discover more about human sexuality yourself—what is fact and what is fallacy: masturbation does not cause warts or blindness; male homosexuals do not wear dresses; old men also wear 'macs' and are usually not 'dirty'; male transvestites are rarely homosexual.

- Be able to show your acceptance of the person's difficulties by helping them without fuss, showing no signs of revulsion at their injuries or hostility to their lifestyle.

- Help people to feel loved, accepted and valued by being with them, especially if they are anxious or distressed; listening, more than talking, is needed to find out what bothers them so that you can seek more expert help for them. Simply being with someone, holding their hand or giving a sincerely affectionate cuddle can all do much to restore an unhappy patient's morale.

It requires considerable sensitivity and knowledge to know how best to help different people in different circumstances. No two people respond to things which affect their sexuality in exactly the same way. Not everyone will find it easy to talk about their feelings on such issues. Much discussion about sexuality was taboo in our culture until quite recently and even now it can be a highly contentious issue. For example the rise of the AIDS problem in the UK and how best to challenge it produced much conflict (and still does). How often should the advertisements be shown on TV? How explicit could they be? Could condoms, words describing homosexual acts or pictures of human sexual organs be shown and openly discussed in the media? Much of the difficulty surrounding the AIDS issue had little to do with the disease itself (the spread of which between carers and patients can be simply prevented by many standard infection control procedures). Rather, the issue relates much more to opinions about sexual expression in our culture, notions of 'good' or 'bad' sex, repressive attitudes to homosexuality and to strongly held beliefs about prostitution, casual sex, drug injection and contraception.

Working as a carer, you have an important role to play in helping someone to express their sexuality. The way in which you help can do much to restore someone's dignity and remove their sense of sexual isolation. If you need to know more, read some of the texts on this issue suggested in the further reading section or contact some of the information centres listed on page 178. Whatever help you give should be given on the basis that you've got your facts right yourself and have come to terms with your own feelings about the issues related to the subject of human sexuality.

12

Resting and sleeping

Sleep has often been referred to as 'the great restorer'. Without it you quickly succumb to feeling weak and drowsy, lacking energy and concentration, being easily confused and mentally unstable.

Most of us establish a regular sleeping pattern which varies very much between individuals. Very small babies spend almost three-quarters of their time asleep, while older adults may feel the need for no more than a few hours each night. The nature of sleep differs too, again from person to person as well as during one episode. It is often described as 'light' or 'heavy' according to how easily the person can be roused from his or her slumbers.

In addition to sleep, everyone takes some form of rest during their waking hours. The rest does not usually take the form of a deep sleep—perhaps just a quiet few moments to yourself with your feet up on the chair and a cup of tea, or perhaps a few moments of solitude on a park bench or lying on the grass. For others the rest period may take the form of a short spell of real sleep or 'nap', perhaps lasting no more than a few minutes.

Whatever its nature, most people sleep regular hours at night with some form of rest period during the day. Rarely, some people have great difficulty sleeping at all (insomnia) or may appear to be drowsy or sleep all day, even to the point of falling asleep frequently (narcolepsy). While the content of this chapter gives advice on helping people to rest and sleep (and for most people these simple points will work well), it is worth remembering that you should seek expert medical advice if sleep becomes either excessive or difficult to achieve.

Healthy people who sleep well wake up feeling more energetic, invigorated and ready to face the day (or night if you are on night duty). People who have health problems, however, need more sleep and rest. This helps the body to concentrate its energies not on physical or mental activity, but on the repair of tissues damaged by injury or infection, or to allow the mind to restore itself after or during particularly stressful times. Promoting rest and sleep are therefore some of the most valuable things you can do to help restore health of body and mind.

Think about the last time you had difficulty getting to sleep. What factors made sleep hard to achieve? Make a list of these and compare with the following.

- Fear
- Anxiety
- Heat
- Cold
- Pain
- Discomfort
- Breathing difficulties
- Effect of some drugs
- Uncomfortable bedclothes
- Position of limbs
- Hunger
- Thirst
- Background noise
- Unfamiliar environment
- Needing to pass urine
- Needing to open bowels
- Loneliness
- Lack of activity
- Lights
- Feeling the need for a wash or bath

The above are some of the things that may reduce your ability to sleep. People who are unwell are likely to experience many of those. Worries about the outcome of an illness or the financial effects on the family can leave the person lying awake and feeling unable to settle. Pains, muscle cramps, 'pins and needles' or just the general discomfort of being in an unfamiliar bed or with insufficient pillows also make rest difficult to achieve. Feeling hungry or thirsty, or wanting to pass urine or open your bowels will prevent sleep, while some drugs we take (even in the form of drinks) such as the caffeine in coffee will tend to keep us awake. Some people find it impossible to sleep with a light on, while others could not sleep without it. If you have not been active during the day you may feel less tired. Any kind of discomfort like feeling too hot or too cold will prevent sleep and any such difficulty seems to loom larger when we are alone in the dark with nothing to distract us.

Most of these difficulties can be fairly and easily overcome in your own home, but ill people who go into hospital or a nursing home have the added stress of trying to sleep in an unfamiliar place with its strange new sounds, other people around them, snoring, nurses walking about and so on.

Take the opportunity to sit quietly at home (if you are nursing at home) or in your place of work. Spend about 10 minutes just listening and looking. What sort of things can you identify in your environment that could limit sleep?

Noise, especially noise that you are unaccustomed to, will prevent or interrupt sleep, while more familiar sounds, however dramatic, may leave us undisturbed.

Sarah had lived all her life by the railway shunting yard. She slept easily despite the nightly noises of clanking carriages and rumbling engines. On holiday she barely slept for three nights, the silence of the cottage was penetrated only by the sound of the sea some way off.

Feeling lonely and vulnerable also contributes to sleeplessness. In hospital you might think that it is difficult to feel lonely, but the environment is full of strangers and unfamiliar and often frightening things. Many people who sleep with a partner may find it hard to sleep in a single bed alone or find it disturbing to be in a room with other people, such as in hospital.

Promoting rest and sleep

There is sometimes a tendency to resort to sedation when rest and sleep are difficult. Perhaps it is better if these methods are kept as the last resort, as the drugs themselves can produce a lot of other problems. There is a great deal you can do as a helper to promote rest and sleep without resort to drugs.

Step one in our strategy is to establish the patient's normal sleep pattern.

To get some idea of the variation in sleep pattern, you could try talking to groups of friends or work colleagues. You will probably find that there is a wide range of sleep patterns in terms of time taken and those who describe themselves as 'heavy' or 'light' sleepers. Try to include some night duty workers and see what they say about their sleep patterns as well.

If you know someone very well you may already be very familiar with his or her normal sleep pattern. If not, you will need to find out from them or their relatives.

Step two is to find the reason for the disruption of this normal sleep pattern. You will need to look very carefully at the factors described above. Look at the environment and the person (and yourself) to assess what might be inhibiting sleep. Are your shoes or the neighbour's noisy? Is the light too bright? Is the person in pain or too hot or too cold?

Step three is to solve the problem. Having identified how someone usually rests and sleeps, and sorted out what might be preventing him or her from doing so, you can set about dealing with the specifics. You may not be able to solve all the difficulties but at least relieving some of them may help the person in need to settle and sleep much better that they would otherwise.

Dealing with worry

You can reassure someone in many simple ways to alleviate anxiety, but it may be that in some circumstances you need to seek expert help, perhaps from your family doctor or community nurse if you are caring for someone at home, or from a trained nurse if you are working in hospital. In the latter case, especially, you need to ensure that details are passed on to the trained staff and you should be wary of getting involved with problems beyond your scope.

You can give much comfort simply by being there, not necessarily speaking, so that the person feels more secure, in the knowledge that he is not alone. In hospital, perhaps you can ensure that a patient who has particular difficulty in sleeping has the use of a single-bed cubicle, or a less busy part of the ward. At the same time, a means of calling you—a nearby bell, call button or telephone—will be helpful.

Be alert to your patient looking anxious or worried, without waiting for him to tell you. Be ready to sit with him and listen to what he has to say. Stay with him if he feels particularly unsettled and try to help him work through the problem, or give information to help to allay his fears. Where you are unable to deal with the problem make sure that your patient is told that you will send someone who can. Remember, old or young, we all derive comfort from physical contact and feel reassured and safer—holding hands or a cuddle can prove very valuable to the anxious and sleepless patient.

Mark is 15 and due to have an operation next day. He tries to put a brave face on it but is really very worried. The doctor has prescribed night sedation, but well before this the nurse spent about 10 minutes talking with him, going over what is to happen and answering his questions. Afterwards he felt and looked more relaxed.

Jack is 69 and is being nursed at home by his wife. Since his 'stroke' he gets alarmed and shouts if he is alone in the room. At night Ethel, his wife, holds his hand and stays with him until he falls asleep.

Promoting relaxation

Helping people to relax can be very important in promoting sleep. Apart from the above features, a few simple techniques can be helpful. For example ask your patient to lie quietly and concentrate on his breathing and to gradually relax all the muscles in his body. Talk to him in a soothing, calm voice and ask him to think of a pleasant scene or event. Thoughts that are soothing or repetitive, like concentrating on breathing, appear to help to induce sleep—the old technique of counting sheep really can help some people!

Many people find a period of reading useful in promoting sleep to relax the mind. Warm drinks or a light supper can be helpful too; but leave large meals or food that the person normally finds difficult to digest.

Drugs might be helpful, but it is probably best to treat these as a last resort. On the other hand, a readily available drug—alcohol—can be a great sleep inducer in small quantities. A glass of beer or sherry last thing at night can produce a warm, relaxed feeling that leads to sleep. Be cautious, however, because excess alcohol can disturb sleep, while it can be positively dangerous with children or when mixed with other drugs—when in doubt consult a doctor or a more senior nurse.

Reducing noise levels

Having satisfied yourself that you have done what you can with your patient to promote sleep, consider next the noise levels that he or she has to cope with. Bear in mind the fact that absolute silence can be just as disturbing as noise, but monitor noise levels carefully and pinpoint sources of irritation. Can a window be closed to reduce noise outside? Does a noisy central heating system prove disturbing? Could a nearby TV be too loud? Check that your own activities as carer are not disturbing your patient:

Start by taking a close look at yourself! Move around the room and listen carefully. What do *you* do that makes noise? Do those shoes clatter, or your clothing rustle? Are you coughing loudly or talking to the person as if he is deaf? Do you bang doors or clatter equipment?

Making the bed more comfortable

It is as well to check the bed for general points of comfort. Run through the following check-list.

- firm mattress or board under mattress for patients with back pain
- free from crumbs and lumps
- sheets crease free, clean and dry
- blankets not too tight or too loose (perhaps a cradle over the foot of the bed to relieve weight of blankets)
- blankets or duvet are warm enough
- sufficient pillows
- perhaps there is a need for a soft or warm under blanket
- big enough (especially for people used to sleeping in large beds)
- are aids such as hot water bottles and electric blankets useful and working?
- are pillows, mattresses, etc, adjustable to support head, back and limbs?

Hospital beds usually have lots of complicated equipment to adjust so that the patient can find the right position. Even without this you can do much to promote comfort, for example with judicious use of support from pillows. This is particularly important where the person has difficulty moving himself—it may be that only you can help him to sleep, simply because he is unable to adjust his position himself. You have probably seen those speeded-up films of people during sleep and noticed how, quite unconsciously, they move around to prevent soreness or poor circulation. Imagine what it is like, lying in one position, desperate to sleep and yet unable to move, while all the time the pain in your back or the 'pins and needles' gets worse. Perhaps you can understand now that the best nurses are those who are not sympathetic but *empathic*, i.e. see a person's problem from his point of view and help him to do something about it. Remember also that many people who are ill find it difficult to sleep in bed (especially those with breathing problems) and a comfortable chair with pillows to support them in an upright position can be just as useful in promoting rest or sleep as the most luxurious bed.

Monitoring the sleep pattern

When in doubt check with your patient. Get him or her to tell you those things which make them more comfortable and what sort of night or nap they have had. If this is not possible, then use your powers of observation to assess how well things have gone. Does your patient look rested and more relaxed? Is his or her breathing easy and colour good? Is he or she free from signs of restlessness or fidgeting? It is part of your caring role to make sure that all that can be done is done; it is equally important to monitor the effectiveness of your treatment.

13

Worshipping

While the number of people attending church in the UK is relatively small and has declined steadily over the years, surveys suggest that most people—over 65%—still regard themselves as 'Christian' when asked their religion. Although Christianity remains the dominant belief system, the history of the UK has led to the presence of many other religions. Immigrants from all parts of the world have brought their beliefs with them, while in the past four hundred years at least, a tolerance of other people's beliefs has become the norm.

Our society is, therefore, not only multiracial, but also multireligious. In considering 'worshipping', therefore, we are looking at a whole range of people's beliefs, from those who deny the existence of any god to those who follow many. Whether you agree or disagree with the patient's beliefs is of little consequence. As a carer, your role is primarily to *accept* his beliefs and not attempt to change him to your own or some other's convictions. Beyond that, you also have another responsibility—to help meet the patient's spiritual needs.

No patient should have his or her religious needs ignored; they are as important to him or her as the help you give with washing or mobilising. When you are unsure, seek advice from a minister of the appropriate religion, from the patient and his or her family or friends and from senior nursing and medical staff.

Practical help

How might you help meet the religious needs in the
following circumstances?

- An elderly lady, housebound, is a devout Catholic and
  used to attending church every week.
- A young man, distressed as his wife is dying, becomes
  angry with you and demands 'why is God letting this
  happen?'
- A child of Jewish parents is in hospital, where all the
  children are non-Jewish.

Perhaps you could discuss these situations with friends or
colleagues.

From these examples, there are a number of practical guidelines
that can be generally applied to helping all people with their worshipping problems. Discussion of the more specific aspects of
some religions will follow later in the chapter.

First, accept the patient's beliefs and feelings for what they are.
When difficulties arise you can refer the patient to an appropriate
minister for guidance.

Second, if you are in a hospital or other such setting, keep a list
of local religious organisations, ministers, etc, and of where they
can be contacted. If in doubt, try the local library, telephone
directory, CAB or a social services office.

Third, it is important to keep yourself up to date with the special practices of various religions so that you do not break what,
for them, could be very important rules. This may be particularly important in relation to diet and certain social taboos.

Fourth, if the patient cannot be taken out to meet the religious
needs (for example to church—you will need to check with a
trained nurse, if appropriate, before you do this), then try and
arrange it so that the religion comes to the patient. Most hospitals have one or more chaplains who will gladly provide religious
services, or can contact others who can provide care for those
with special needs. It may even occur that the patient asks you to
share his religious rituals with him—to pray with him for example. There is no reason why you should not do this if it provides

comfort to your patient and if you feel that you can participate honestly and sincerely. If not, then you will need to tactfully and politely decline. On the other hand it may simply be that he would like your company while he prays.

Fifth, privacy is often an important part of many religious rites. While peace, solitude and a private room may be achievable at home, in hospital or nursing home, this may be rather more difficult. Usually there is some way that this can be arranged—making temporary use of a quiet part of the ward for example, screening off a few beds or using a treatment room that is not needed for a little while. A 'do not disturb' notice on the door can be a good idea to avoid interruptions. A trained nurse should supervise the organisation of ward services.

Finally, it is worth remembering that religion also has a social as well as a personal dimension. While at home or in hospital it may be possible to bring small groups of people of similar beliefs together, either for a chat or for a formal service. Hospitals, hospices and so on which have their own places of worship, are often multidenominational, providing a peaceful setting which people of any religion can use with out offence.

Some specific religious practices

It would be impossible to cover all information on this aspect in the space available here, but a few major points are given for your guidance. When in doubt, of course, the best method is to ask the patient, his relatives or other carers what his special needs are and how you might help. You will probably find that learning about other people's beliefs, especially the less well known ones, would bring added interest to your own work. In addition, it provides a source of conversation to add to the knowledge of each other that is necessary in the caring relationship between you and your patient.

Christianity

The various Christian denominations have at their core a belief in one god and the life of Jesus Christ as the son of God. There are, however, variations in the way different sects approach illness or dying.

The *Church of England* (C of E) emphasises penitence (a desire to repent for sins), charity (goodwill, honesty, love towards others) and strength of faith. Many people prefer to have their minister with them as death approaches.

Roman Catholic (RC) beliefs lay considerable emphasis upon reconciliation and absolution for the forgiveness of sins. If illness becomes more serious then the 'sacrament of the sick' is offered (formerly known as the 'last rites'). The main aim is to offer strength, support and consolation. This is not necessarily a private experience and relatives, carers and other patients may join in if wished. While the priest's presence may be requested as death approaches, to offer prayers and support to the patient and his relatives, it is not essential if the sacrament has been given and anyone may read the prayers provided for the dying person.

The Free Church is a term which embodies the many Christian sects outside the two main orders (C of E and R C) There are no specific rituals for illness or death, but it is worth noting that prayer and communion services are a strong celerient in these faiths.

Some of the Christian faiths have dietary requirements, e.g. abstinence from alcohol, or avoiding meat at varying times of year. You will need to check with your patient for his particular preferences.

Judaism

Orthodox Jews have strict dietary control (no meat from the pig, certain fasting days, etc) and have rituals in relation to the preparation of food (for example meat and milk foods must be kept apart in cooking and eating and animals are ritually slaughtered). Foods prepared according to Jewish law are called 'kosher' foods. There are other practices in relation to the hair and the men prefer beards. Circumcision for boys eight days after birth is customary. Some *liberal Jews* have slight modification to these rules and it is important to know what your patient's preferences are. At death, the presence of the rabbi and family is preferred, any of whom may say prayers. After death the nurses are allowed to close the patient's eyes, tie up the jaw and straighten the limbs.

Hinduism

Hindus worship many gods and goddesses. The cow is considered sacred and therefore practising Hindus will not eat beef. Most female Hindus would not accept a male doctor or nurse for close contact or examination. The presence of the Hindu priest (pandit) is preferred as death approaches and the body is usually washed and prepared afterwards by relatives.

Islam

Muslims must pray to Allah five times each day, preferably using a prayer mat on the ground. However, sitting in a chair or in bed is acceptable. The Muslim teacher will visit in illness or at death, when the patient's feet must point south-east so that he or she faces Mecca. The family will prepare the body after death and it should not be touched by hospital staff.

Meat from pigs is not eaten and there is a period of fasting at Ramadan (but ill patients and women menstruating or after childbirth are exempt). It is worth noting that for both *Hindus* and *Muslims* avoidance of pig meat includes items contaminated by them (frying pans, kitchen surfaces, etc, as well as drugs such as porcine insulin, which is extracted from pigs).

Hindus and *Muslims* also prefer to wash in free flowing water, including after using the toilet, rather than using toilet paper. Showers or a running tap are preferred to a bath or sink of water. Modesty is also important for women. In some cases, male medical and nursing staff would not be acceptable except in emergency, and they require single sex wards. Clothing is expected to maintain modesty, covering the body down to the ankles. Many male Moslems may not accept help or instruction from female nurses or doctors. If difficulties arise you will need to consult a senior nurse.

Buddhism

Buddhists lay particular emphasis on meditation and will need quiet intervals at certain times of the day. Again, you will need to determine the patient's preferences. Vegetarianism is common and the presence of a Buddhist monk in illness and as death approaches is comforting.

14

Dying and bereavement

Death eventually comes to us all—it is the only certainty in life and as we age we are expected to come to terms with our own mortality. We must learn to accept and prepare for it.

At the beginning of this century, death was an everyday part of community life. Childbirth was dangerous and many women in labour and their newborn babies died. Life expectancy was shorter as diseases spread and killed many; only with the development of antibiotics in the 1940s did the infection rate reduce. The First World War contributed to the death rate at home and abroad; work places were hazardous and unclean; there was no state provision for care. Before the birth of the NHS in 1948 many terminally ill patients were nursed in their own homes. Families stayed close, living in the same area and able to give family support, so death was an event most families experienced.

Nowadays, with improved medical techniques, greater life expectancy and increased opportunity to be nursed in hospitals, we can go through our lives never dealing with grief or loss due to death. The Centre for Policy on Ageing (CPA) undertook a survey in 1983 and found that 70% of deaths in urban areas took place in hospital.

No one can prepare you for the emotions you may feel when a patient you have cared for dies. You may have looked after the patient for some time before he or she dies and grown to like both patient and relatives. Therefore it is only natural for you to feel unhappiness at his death and sadness for the relatives. Many years ago, the nursing profession frowned upon this involvement with patients and their families; nowadays it is accepted and understood. However, your sadness should not make you incapable of looking after your other patients and your grief should not affect your home or your social life. If you do feel emotionally stressed do not hesitate to talk to your nursing sister. Do not try to cope on your own.

Death may be accidental, at home, on the road or at work, or it may be caused by a sudden illness like a stroke (CVA) or heart attack (myocardial infarction). Alternatively, death may be the end of a chronic illness such as cancer, heart, kidney or lung disease. No matter what the cause of death, the effects of the loss can be devastating to the relatives and those close to the patient. As a carer you will have to come to terms with what is, after all, a natural progression from life.

Terminally ill patients do not necessarily need to be bed-ridden; they may only become dependent towards the end when they become weaker. There are many stages of physical dependence prior to death and the aims of caring will change as the patient's needs change.

Control of pain

One of the most important responsibilities you have will be to observe for pain. It can breed fear and, in turn, fear can cause tension and increase pain. The patient may tell you that he or she is in pain but many patients *fear* that increasing levels of pain-killers (analgesics) may make them unable to function mentally and they will not wish for their remaining time with their loved ones to be blurred. Therefore they may try to cope with the pain. Patients in pain may look uncomfortable or find it difficult to move. If you believe the patient is in pain, or if he or she tells you so, you must inform the nurse in charge *immediately*. Recently, pain control has become extremely efficient. It is now possible to alleviate pain without 'blurring' the patient's mental state.

Comfort

Your second responsibility is to keep the patient comfortable. This involves positioning your patient comfortably and, by so doing, protecting skin and pressure areas (see Chapter 4). The use of various pressure relieving aids, such as ripple mattresses, sheepskins and bootees, will help *but* these are *only* aids. The real preventative treatment will always be regular turning of the patient. If there are pressure relieving aids in use your responsibility extends to making sure that all are in good working order and any faults or defects are reported immediately. Many patients will not be comfortable nursed in bed and may prefer to be nursed in a chair or, if at home, on a settee. This should be possible to arrange with permission from the nursing staff. In one hospice a patient was kept comfortable by giving him regular warm baths. Comfort also includes personal cleanliness, so long as it is not at the expense of creating more pain. Allow the patient to tell you what would give comfort.

The same principles for bathing apply to the terminally ill patient; it will help morale but you should always remember that as much as possible the patient should be allowed to attend to his or her own personal hygiene.

Sometimes terminally ill patients experience a sudden rapid rise in body temperature followed by a sudden fall as sweating occurs (rigors). They will feel fresher after sponging but at such times they may also feel exhausted. Use your observation skills to establish what would be best for the patient—sleep or attention to hygiene.

Some terminally ill patients may have jaundice. This is a yellowish tinge of the skin produced by the waste products in the blood. It can produce an irritating itch which the patient may believe will be relieved by washing. This, however, is not the case and you should inform the nurse in charge, as certain medication from the doctor can help to relieve this unpleasant symptom.

An area that is sometimes sadly neglected is the patient's mouth. If the patient has problems with eating or drinking, due to nausea or vomiting, he or she will become dehydrated. One of the symptoms of dehydration is a dry, coated tongue. Your responsibility is to alleviate such conditions and help to keep the mouth moist and fresh. The best way is by using a toothbrush and toothpaste or by removing dentures regularly and using mouthwashes. If your patient cannot swallow, or has a sore mouth, ask the nurse to provide a mouth care pack which contains special swabs which can be used instead of a brush.

How does your mouth feel when you have been ill and have not eaten for a day or two? Imagine this continuing for even longer.

If your patient's mouth is merely dry then ice cubes can be a pleasant way of relieving dryness. You can obtain mouthwashes from the local chemist and carbonated drinks have been found to promote mouth freshness.

Diet and elimination

Some patients may find it difficult to eat or drink due to nausea or vomiting. At these times a light, semi-soft diet may be tolerated and this can be made with a liquidiser. If the patient does not have access to one, it may be possible to obtain one for hire from Cancer Relief, Cripples' Help Society (see page 179) or perhaps local charities.

Fluid intake is of the utmost importance as this will help keep the body's minerals balanced and keep the kidneys in working order. In hospitals, an intravenous infusion (drip) may be put into the patient's arm or hand to restore fluid balance. In such cases, you must ensure that the arm is kept supported at all times and that the bandages are never wet (this will mean that the infusion has become disconnected). You must also note the condition of the arm above and below the bandage and report any redness, heat or inflammation.

If the patient is being nursed in bed or is attached to an intravenous infusion (IVI), it may be necessary to use a commode and/or urinals and bedpans.

In most hospitals there are now papier mâché bedpans and urinals which are more hygienic and more comfortable for the patient. However, in the patient's own home plastic bedpans and urinals or commodes can be borrowed from the local health centres for the patient's own use.

With many terminally ill patients, the bowels become sluggish and can result in constipation, not only because of the illness but perhaps also dehydration, immobility and some types of medication. You will have to report your fears to the nurse in charge and a plan for relief of constipation will be formulated. You may be asked to increase the patient's intake of fluids and you must record how much is being taken. Aperients (laxatives) may be given on doctor's instruction and an enema may also help to relieve this unpleasant condition.

In some cases, the patient may have diarrhoea; this in itself is unpleasant but it can lead to extremely sore areas around the anus. This can be prevented and treated with a regular application of a barrier cream such as zinc and castor oil after gentle washing and drying.

Finally you must be most diligent about the hygienic care of catheters (see Chapter 7). Any redness or soreness around the end of the penis in men and the urethral opening in women should be reported immediately. You should also make sure that the catheter is draining satisfactorily and that there is no blood or sediment in the catheter bag.

Having taken care of the physical comforts of the patient there is much you can do to help the patient psychologically. Talking to your patient, giving your time for a chat is a precious activity and will help the patient by distracting him or her for a short period. You can also help with any other recreational activity he or she would like to do, such as crosswords, reading and letter writing.

Other help available

Home help service

In certain circumstances, for example an elderly infirm couple or a terminally ill patient living alone or with an elderly partner, a 'home help' can be arranged from the social services department. He or she will clean and tidy the house and perhaps do some shopping (in some areas a small fee is charged).

Meals on wheels

For a nominal charge, the social services will arrange for a hot midday meal to be delivered to the patient's own home but, unfortunately, they are unable to provide special or semi-soft diets.

Laundry service

In some areas, a domiciliary service is available, whereby used or soiled sheets, pillow cases and nightwear are collected and clean ones delivered once a week. Check with the nurse if this service runs in your area.

Night sitters (Marie Curie nurses)

Some patients can be quite restless during the evening and in the night and may therefore need 24-hour care. Relatives will need help and support to cope with such a task. Marie Curie nurses are specially trained and obtainable in certain areas to sit with the patient at night, allowing the relatives to get some necessary sleep. This is especially valuable to relatives under stress or as the patient's condition worsens.

Emotional care

You may be caring for a patient who is unaware of how seriously ill he or she is. The relatives may not want the patient to be told the true seriousness of the illness. Perhaps they have in the past discussed whether or not he or she wishes to be told or it may be a family decision without the patient's knowledge. Whatever decision has been made, *you* must *respect* it. This can be difficult to accept, especially if the patient asks you the question 'Am I going to die?'. Many care assistants and auxilliaries often worry about what they would say if a patient asks this question. If the situation ever arises, and that is unlikely, it will perhaps make it easier for you if you have explored your answer prior to the question.

No one will ask you to tell an outright lie to the patient so a standard answer may be the best solution both for your patient and yourself: 'I do not know all the details of your illness but the sister will be able to give you an informed answer and, as it obviously worries you, would you like me to ask her to talk to you about it?'

Many patients come to terms with the knowledge that they are dying and want to arrange their own affairs, but you must remember it is the decision of the family, nurses and doctors whether they should be told.

Religion appears to play a major part in the way some people come to terms with death. Even those who have never had faith can get comfort from religion towards the end of their illness and may request to see the clergy. Another important aspect of a person's life is their culture; it will be important that their cultural rites are adhered to *especially* at this time.

All patients who know that they are dying will experience certain stages of emotion, which are part of the natural process of grief for themselves and the patient has to go through them in accepting his own death. You should be aware of these emotions and try not to be shocked by their display:

- The patient may initially be shocked at the news, become quiet, withdrawn and solemn.
- Next, there may be an outburst of anger, which can be aimed at themselves or their loved ones or those around him (including nurses). Understand that this is not a personal attack and explain this to the relatives.
- This process may be followed by disbelief, guilt and depression before all concerned are able to accept the diagnosis.

In 1985 The British Association of Cancer United Patients (BACUP) was formed (a new support organisation for cancer patients and their loved ones). This helps people to go through their grieving process and links people with a certain type of cancer to others who have been through the same experience. BACUP also gives practical advice and information on many problems facing the cancer patients and their families, as well as running a telephone service offering counselling or just a friendly chat (see page 178).

Finally, remember that to die is the last experience an individual can go through and it is therefore hardly surprising that many wish to be *in control* of the way in which they spend their last few months, weeks or even days. Your responsibility is to allow the patient's end to be as dignified as possible. If you treat the patient as an individual with specific needs and choices and if you respect them, you will help maintain their dignity at this vital time.

Hospices

For patients who can no longer be cared for at home there is an alternative to hospital care: Dame Cecily Saunders founded the hospices for terminally ill patients and their relatives to come to terms with approaching death in a peaceful, pain-free and spiritually tranquil setting. Nowadays, we have hospices in most areas of Britain and although most people tend to be reluctant to go to them initially, once they have experienced the comfort and cheerfulness of the properly trained staff and their efforts to relieve pain, they are happy to return. Once the pain is controlled, the patient and his or her loved ones are free to face the future as rationally as possible in tranquil settings.

Nurses in hospices are taught the importance of giving patients time to talk about their fears and patients are encouraged to ask questions. Sometimes there are no answers to be given but the patient will feel the need to ask the question anyway.

At the present time there is a move to take the aims and objectives of hospice care away from institutions and into the patient's home, with the help of specially trained district nurses.

Last offices

However well prepared you are to care for a terminally ill patient you will of course be upset when he or she dies. You will understandably be apprehensive about assisting with attending to the person who has just died, but it may be made easier for you if you bear in mind what an experienced ward sister once said to me when I was a student nurse:

'This is the last caring act you can do for your patient'. It is also a time for you to say goodbye to your patient and to bring comfort to those relatives left behind. Always observe specific religious or cultural requirements before performing the last offices. For example for *Roman Catholic* patients the ritual of the last sacrament must be performed by the priest and this ritual is still valid after death; for *Christian Scientists* female patients should be 'laid out' by females.

Remember that if there are communication problems between the relatives and the nursing staff, interpreters can be obtained in most health authorities, and their help may be very important at this sad time.

The following is a broad guide to hospital procedure, although it may differ from hospital to hospital.

As with all procedures, prepare all your equipment before-hand on a trolley.

- The body should be washed and dried thoroughly.
- Any wounds should have new large dressings applied securely (including pressure sores).
- The hair should be combed.
- Most health authorities suggest that false teeth should be replaced in the mouth (check with the nurse in charge).
- The limbs should be straightened.
- The patient should be dressed in a shroud.
- The patient should have an arm/leg band noting name, age, religion, hospital number, date and ward. (There are alternative ways of labelling (check with the nurse in charge).
- A sheet should be placed under and over the patient.
- All personal property should be listed and any valuables placed in the ward safe.

Many relatives and close friends may wish to see their dead relative or friend. Death can be an end to suffering and in cases like this the patient often looks at peace, but death can also be traumatic and the patient may look unlike him/herself. The nurse in charge must be made aware of visiting relatives and will then talk to them. Seeing the body of a loved one who has died can help the relatives come to terms with the death, say goodbye and face reality.

Your role will be to tidy the area around the bedside, removing all unnecessary equipment, etc. The bedside locker should be cleared and perhaps some flowers placed upon it. You may be asked to stay with the relatives or to make them a drink.

Grief is a natural emotion and one you may be personally

familiar with. If not you must not be shocked by what you see or hear. Some people are reserved in grief and may sob quietly; others may shout and cry loudly and some may remain silent. You may experience different reactions and different ethnic races and cultures have their own way of showing grief.

Personal touch at this time is most reassuring. A gentle hand on the grieving visitor's shoulder or arm may help. If there is silence do not let it embarrass you, instead respect that individual's need for silence.

Grief will continue long after the relatives have left the hospital or, if death occurred at home, long after you have gone. The bereaved partner will probably grieve the most of all the relatives. He or she will experience loneliness, missing not only the person but also perhaps the social settings they used to enjoy together, such as the public house, theatre, library, shops, etc. Everything they do, everywhere they go and perhaps everyone they meet will remind them of their partner in some way or other. They may dream day and night that their partner is still with them, then awake and face the reality of the situation once again. Death is the biggest change in the lives of the remaining partners. Bereaved husbands not only have grief for their loss but also have to come to terms with the day to day tasks of running a house, something he may well have not experienced fully so far in his life.

There are many voluntary organisations (see page 178) that may be able to help the grieving relative and it may be useful to remember these organisations when you finally visit the relative after the death.

You as a carer will be helping to care not only for the terminally ill patient, but also his family. Remember this when you attend to the patient and spend some time talking to the relatives; they will appreciate it. They may also wish to help care for their relative, and this should be encouraged as it will make them feel more useful and perhaps less frustrated. Remember also that they know the patient's likes and dislikes.

Death has to be accepted by our society as inevitable and we must all learn to talk more openly about it, for eventually we will all have to accept it and prepare for it.

15

Caring for the sick child

In order to understand best how to care for the sick child, we need to understand the normal development of the child from infancy, through childhood, up to and including adolescence. Child development is a vast subject and at times a complicated one. The aim of this brief review of the subject is to demonstrate to you the value of understanding child development when applied to giving care to this section of the population.

Infancy (0-5 years)

Having lived in the warm and protective environment of the womb, the newborn infant must rapidly adjust to life in the outside world. Immediate needs are oxygen, nourishment, human contact, warmth and rest. Breathing accomplished, the newborn child next seeks nourishment and within hours a regular feeding pattern is normally established. Simultaneously, a loving relationship begins to form between mother and baby, known as the bonding process. From the age of six weeks this relationship is further enhanced as the baby is able to recognise his or her mother.

Temperature control and the ability to maintain a normal body temperature, i.e. 37 degrees centigrade (37°C) is poor in the infant. *Hypothermia*, a condition where the body temperature falls below 35°C, can rapidly develop in very young babies. As elimination at this stage of development is an uncontrolled action, frequent changing is necessary if heat loss is to be avoided. Care is also required, when bathing the baby, to ensure the bath water is kept at body temperature. Conversely, a high body temperature, above 37.5°C (a condition known as *pyrexia*) can quickly result from overclothing the baby, or from prolonged bouts of crying. Care should be taken to avoid both events.

Keeping the baby's environment free of *infection* is essential. The single most important measure in preventing infection reaching the baby, is *effective* handwashing, prior to handling the baby or preparing his feed. The skin is an important barrier to infection, and as a baby is easily damaged, extreme care should be taken when handling the baby. The baby's eyes are also very vulnerable to infection as the blinking reflex and the tear glands do not work efficiently in early life. Special care must be taken if the baby is born prematurely.

From around the age of two months the infant begins to influence his own development through *communication*. He can convey pleasure by smiling and gurgling, or displeasure by frowning or crying. As his brain develops he becmes capable of more complex forms of communication, laughing and, later, language. The infant who is continually talked to will respond by trying to imitate the sounds he hears. Learning to talk is one of the most fascinating achievements of early life.

Infancy is a period of rapid *growth* and as a result it is essential that the infant receives the correct nourishment and obtains adequate rest. With growth comes *strength* and, from strength, *mobility*. By the age of eight months he can sit up unsupported, by nine months he is crawling. Walking unaided is achieved by the age of 13 months. Getting up and down stairs and jumping are perfected by the age of 18 months, and by two years he is able to run!

As the child's strength and mobility increases so does his power of *manipulation*. The ability to feed himself is one of the first manipulative skills to be mastered at around 15 months of age. By the age of two years he is able to dress himself. It is all too easy to stifle this process of independence. The carer may be tempted to feed the child herself and save time cleaning up the mess afterward. Similarly, to dress the child herself, rather than allow the child, through experience, to learn the correct order in which to button up his coat. It may save time initially but will keep the child dependent.

From the second year onwards the child gains *control over elimination*. Control over defecation is achieved first. The time to start toilet training depends on each individual child's readiness. One of the first indicators of readiness is the child becoming aware of a full bladder.

The need for love is fundamental. From a stable and close relationship in infancy, the child can grow with self-confidence and a feeling of self-worth. Much of a child's behaviour is concerned with seeking acceptance and approval: children love to please and, in turn, to be praised and loved.

Most of the child's time in infancy has been spent learning to become independent within a small social world, one comprising mainly of his home life and family. It is not until going to nursery and later to school that he significantly extends his knowledge of the kind of society in which he lives. Much of the next stage of development—childhood—is spent developing this awareness of the world around him.

Childhood (6–12 years)

As the child moves into school, physically the rate and amount of growth is considerably less dramatic than that seen in infancy. Although individual variations in size become more apparent, so do the physical differences between the sexes later in childhood.

The child continues to perfect skills already begun, for example motor development; this is made possible by the child's increasing mastery over speed and strength. Co-operative games become an important feature of the social interaction that takes place within this age group. These games demand a high degree of speed, strength, agility, co-ordination and precision from those participating.

Play is the most important single means by which children increase their knowledge of the world around them and learn what is, and what is not, socially acceptable behaviour. For instance playing with toys teaches the child the importance of respect for material things. Co-operative play teaches the child some of the values of life such as competitiveness and sharing.

In most societies with a formal education system, the child now attends *school* full-time where he learns the complex skills of reading, writing, spelling, formal language and counting. Verbal skills are further developed with an increased vocabulary and fluency of speech. Some children learn more quickly than others and differences in terms of the ability to learn become apparent through the competitiveness that exists within education itself.

The child's *emotional development* is no longer solely under the influence of his parents and family. He now has a group of friends and school teachers to affect his development. The child still relies heavily on his parents for encouragement and praise and, although increasingly self-reliant, still needs comforting and protection from sources of fear and anxiety. His parents also continue to influence his social behaviour, emotional development and feeling of self-worth. In addition they affect the moral standards he will carry into the next stage of development, adolescence and beyond.

During infancy the child was made aware of his *sexuality* by society's expectations of the norm, i.e. what is 'boyish' behaviour or is not. In childhood the child becomes aware of his own sexuality, taking pleasure in his body. Often he models himself upon the parent of the same sex.

Although a young child misses his parents if separated from them, he can cope with temporary separation, because he now has the ability to understand time, reasoning and promises.

The greatest amount of development in childhood takes place in *social development*. The child's life becomes less family dominated. School friends provide opportunities for co-operation and competition, and the child usually associates with a number of different peer groups as well as adult neighbours, each group providing social relationships of various strengths and types. Within each of these groups the child will learn more of the 'rules of life'; for example, trust and responsibility for others and in today's multiracial society, respect for other cultures and lifestyles.

From time to time most children have to face periods of unhappiness and anxiety; childhood is not without its problems, however trivial they may seem to adults. The loss of a family pet, never mind a grandparent, can be a very distressing event for a child; handled correctly it can enrich emotional development.

On the whole, most children are protected from the responsibilities and obligations of adulthood during these early years. The time is spent learning about the society in which they live. In the last stage of development—adolescence—the child's task is to assume a place in that society.

Adolescence (13–18 years)

The time of adolescence—the passing from childhood to maturity—is less easily definable in today's society. Whilst the right to vote heralds the end of adolescence, other cultures within our society cite sexual maturity as the entry into adulthood.

Physical development in adolescence is dominated by the development of secondary sexual characteristics the onset being called *puberty*. Unfortunately, emotional development is not achieved until some time later, leaving the poor adolescent feeling awkward and confused, especially when in the company of the opposite sex.

In the female, the first signs of puberty, which can occur at any time from the age of eight years (but usually happens around the age of 12 years) are enlargement of the breasts and growth of pubic hair. In addition, the hips widen and fat deposits are laid down, which gives rise to the characteristic female shape. At the same time the abdominal organs enlarge, particularly those of the reproductive system. Physical maturity is reached with the onset of menstruation, said to occur around the age of 13 years but often earlier.

Males tend to reach puberty slightly later than females. Characteristically there is an increase in body size and muscle power and a decrease in the amount of baby fat, or 'puppy fat' as it is commonly called. Changes within the body, in relation to physical growth also occur: the blood pressure rises, heart rate falls, blood volume increases and respiratory efficiency improves. The age at which these changes take place varies and can be a cause of further anxiety in the male adolescent. Growth of the sex organs, the appearance of body and facial hair and the deepening of the voice mark the arrival of sexual maturity and the completion of physical development.

The adolescent's *emotional development* is closely related to the physical changes of puberty. Although physically equal to an adult, the adolescent has not yet acquired the emotional ability to cope with the responsibilities and obligations of adulthood. This leads to conflict; relationships with parents undergo change and the adolescent begins to assert his or her individuality and desire for independence by resisting adult authority. Adolescence is often a period of emotional turmoil; the conflict lies between the adolescent's desire for independence and his or her need for the security of childhood. This results in mood swings and confused emotions. The adolescent is capable of being both happy and miserable, full of energy one moment and lazy the next.

The *formal educational system* remains a feature of adolescent life and the level of achievement between individuals shows an even more marked differentiation between individual achievements than in childhood; while some achieve advanced examinations, others fail to reach an acceptable standard of literacy and numeracy.

Social development is rapid and the adolescent's social world expands rapidly. Boys tend to reinforce their masculinity and channel their physical energies by grouping together and engaging in sports or other male activities. Girls tend to become concerned with their physical appearance and femininity and their associations with each other are often competitive rather than co-operative and friendly.

Later in adolescence boy/girl relationships become common and although often transient, can be intense and traumatic; often adolescents indulge in some degree of sexual experimentation; occasionally they can develop into permanent adult relationships. Unfortunately the inherent risk of sexual experimentation is the occurrence of an unwanted pregnancy despite the widespread availability of contraceptive devices. A far more common problem is that of becoming dependent for life on drugs, such as nicotine, alcohol or heroin; a habit formed in adolescence is very hard to break.

Reactions to illness and hospitalisation

No one is suggesting for a moment that any normal child looks forward to hospital attendance or enjoys being ill. However, whether that period of hospitalisation has a positive or negative effect in terms of the child's emotional development will depend largely on the consideration shown to him by those involved in his care.

The hospital is an unfamiliar and imposing structure with strange rooms, equipment, sounds and people in 'funny clothes'. For a child who is already feeling frightened and vulnerable through accident or illness, being thrust into this bewildering environment is the final insult. The youngster with imagination can transform 'our' familiar surroundings into a world where drip-stands are 'stick men' with spaghetti tube arms to hold you tightly; the bleep of the ECG (electrocardiogram) monitor is a Martian's ray gun and strange people with no mouths and white coats whisk you away in the middle of the night. For most of us it is difficult to remember what it was like to see the world through the eyes of a child. Obviously, a child's reaction to traumatic events will be dependent on many factors, not least of all his personality, age, previous experience and parental preparation.

In this section we consider the more common behavioural responses of children to illness and hospitalisation in relation to the three age divisions introduced at the beginning of the chapter. It must be stressed, however, that each child is an individual and behaviour is therefore likely to differ accordingly.

The infant is normally relaxed, happy and content as long as his or her needs for warmth, food and comfort are met. When he or she is subjected to restraint, painful stimuli or improper feeding, increasingly vigorous physical emotional activity is observed. The baby is likely to struggle in a vain attempt to withdraw from what 'troubles' him, and unless the comfort he seeks is provided, tension and frustration will increase.

The capacities for memory and anticipation begin in the first few months of life. This is clearly demonstrated in special care nurseries where babies will cry when being held in a particular way, in anticipation of pain.

All babies have the need for emotional satisfaction and when very young they are indiscriminate regarding its source. It is very important that, whenever possible, the mother is resident with her sick baby to promote bonding. Here the role of the care assistant is to help her provide all the normal infant care required, both physical and emotional. Babies deprived of normal stimulation and affection become passive and unresponsive, making it more difficult for the mother to cope with her baby once home.

Probably the most 'difficult' children to cope with in hospital are the toddlers and pre-school children. The normal child of this age protests loudly at being brought to hospital (unless severely ill), and will prove difficult to console when parents leave for home. Understanding is still immature enough to render 'adult' explanations ineffective; while he is quite categorical about his parents' identity—no one else will do!

Responses to separation may take the form of temper tantrums, refusal of food or vomiting. This behaviour is a natural consequence of the child's self-assertiveness and dislike of disruption of his or her routine. Perhaps the child to be more concerned about is the one who is excessively passive and withdrawn or, conversely, gregarious and indiscriminate in his search for affection. This may be indicative of the adverse effects of repeated hospital admissions, separation from his family and exposure to large numbers of strangers, or it could be a sign of adult family tensions. Further investigation into the cause is very important, with the guidance and support of the trained paediatric nurse.

A child of school age has, by now, a wider experience of life both within and away from his family. This may mean greater adaptability to new situations. His degree of understanding is such that he requires a more 'adult' explanation of his predicament. Nevertheless, in times of stress regression in behaviour does occur and he will still need the presence and support of his parents.

Although the child will undoubtedly be distressed by the prospect of painful or unpleasant procedures, it is of paramount importance not to withhold such information or, worse still, lie about impending events. There must be trust within the relationships between child, parents and care giver.

Adolescence is frequently characterised by defiance of authority figures and strivings for independence. These needs do not cease when illness intervenes, thus creating a likely source of frustration and anger when they are thwarted. Hospital staff and parents may be regular recipients of direct or indirect expression of these negative feelings. To the adolescent, hospital care often represents an invasion of privacy and an imposition, resulting in rejection of offers of help, comfort or sympathy.

How to aid adjustment to sickness

One of the main ways to reduce distressed behaviour in the young child is to reduce the length of separation from his or her family—particularly the mother. This can be achieved through unrestricted visiting or provision for resident parents if other family commitments allow. Failing that, the young child needs consistent handling, preferably by a limited number of staff to promote the development of a trusting relationship.

The child should be allowed to keep a favourite toy with him; this helps to maintain the bond with home and is often an invaluable source of comfort. In addition, parents may wish to leave an item of theirs with the child when they leave the ward, thus reassuring him of their return. If parents have been in the habit of saying 'I'm just away to the toilet', when they are in fact, going home, they should be dissuaded from doing so. While dishonesty prevents them from witnessing their child's distress, it is likely to cause feelings of mistrust and insecurity.

If the child is not too unwell it may be appropriate to encourage dressing in his normal clothes. This will help decrease his feelings of vulnerability as opposed to 'stripping' him of his identity when placed in a hospital gown. If this is impracticable then his own night attire or brightly coloured hospital pyjamas or nightdresses are preferable.

When temper tantrums and disruptive behaviour are the prominent feature, measures must be taken to calm the child. This is perhaps one of the most difficult things to do, for it is one's natural reaction to sympathise with a sick child and pander to his needs more than usual. However, no constraints on a child's behaviour, far from giving him freedom of expression, increase his feelings of insecurity and lack of control. The parents should be helped to fulfil this aspect of their role in a positive manner, as they would do under normal circumstances. It may be that they feel they cannot chastise their child, particularly if he is severely ill or dying. Understanding and empathy are very important, and staff may be able to demonstrate that in some cases a firm approach is rewarding.

The withdrawn child's needs can be easily forgotten in a busy paediatric ward. Again, if the presence of a close relative is impossible to arrange, then sensitive handling by a limited number of staff is best. As a care assistant you are likely to be called upon to help by devoting time and patience to this child's social and emotional needs. You are more likely to form a trusting relationship than nursing staff with whom the child may associate unpleasant experiences.

In caring for the older child and adolescent the single most important factor in their care is to respect their privacy and dignity. They may prefer the facilities of a single room so that they can make it their den with articles that they have brought from home. Relating to them in a thoughtful and adult manner is likely to ease adjustment and promote mutual respect.

Play

Play is a vital part of child development, not merely a means of learning the skills of daily living but also a source of pleasure, experimentation and socialisation. For the sick child, at home or in hospital, play has additional benefits in its therapeutic value, allowing expression of fear, anger and frustration. Play is also a medium through which parents and staff can explain unpleasant events during hospitalisation.

As a care assistant you will find that much of your time will be spent providing play for the sick child, in conjunction with nursery nurses and play leaders. Table 15.1 provides suggestions of suitable toys and activities and shows how their benefits can be maximised.

Specific help or advice should be sought from the child's parents or the paediatric nurses with whom you work. A further useful source is the Toy Libraries Association, the address of which is on page 181.

Table 15.1 Toys and play activities for the sick child

Age group	Toy or play activity	Value	Therapeutic use
Late infancy and childhood	Water	Relaxation Imaginative play — bathing dolls, tea parties, etc Encourages use of fine movement: pouring accurately Teaches relationship between size and volume	Reduces tension, anxiety Boisterous water play is an outlet for aggression Continues basic education Main use by ambulant children in play area
	Sand	Tactile stimulation Pleasant association for child: seaside Constructive play: making sand castles Use of hand/eye co-ordination	Use for child with visual impairment — he can enjoy the 'feel' of sand Destroying castles is an outlet for frustration Main use by ambulant children because of practicalities
Childhood	Dough or plasticine	Creative play: making models, cakes, etc Use of manipulative skills	Improves concentration Suitable for most age groups Helps to strengthen 'grip' in child's hands (for example when arm newly removed from plaster cast) Used by child confined to bed

Table 15.1 *Continued*

Age group	Toy or play activity	Value	Therapeutic use
Late infancy and childhood	Building bricks/ wooden shapes	Fosters hand/eye co-ordination Language development: name shapes and colours	Improves ability to grasp objects Identification by touch alone in child with visual impairment
Infancy	Mobiles	Provides environmental stimulation Movement with music — soothing for an infant Encourages eye fixation	Help to prevent sensory deprivation Encourages attentiveness and mobility in young children
Infancy childhood and adolescence	Soft toys and dolls	Tactile value — comforting Expression of affection Use in imaginative play	Bond with home maintained Children of all ages have a doll or soft toy that they like to keep with them Child can act out unpleasant procedures, such as giving an injection, on 'teddy' Staff may use dolls to explain unfamiliar, things to a child

Childhood	Clothes and hospital equipment	Dramatic play	Encourages social contact with other children: 'Doctors and Nurses'; 'Mummys and Daddys'	Helps child relive happy events or come to terms with unhappy events
				Reduces child's loneliness
				Helps to make unfamiliar equipment such as stethoscopes less frightening
Childhood and adolescence	Painting/visual arts	Use of fine motor skills		Useful for child confined to bed
		Encourages creativity		Improves concentration and co-ordination
		Emphasises sense of achievement		Useful outlet for emotional expression, particularly in adolescence. Pleasant memory of hospital to take home with child

The demands of caring for sick children

Caring for sick children is extremely rewarding, but not without its demands and often the arousal of strong emotions which need to be controlled to be beneficial. For example it is easy to feel anger towards a parent who had 'battered' their child; naturally we want to protect those who are vulnerable and defenceless. These feelings should be discussed with trained staff on the unit, social worker or chaplain so that a level of understanding can be reached.

Caring for the dying child and his or her family is also emotionally demanding, requiring compassion and sensitivity when we ourselves may be in need of support. Withdrawal from the situation protects staff but helps no one, whereas over-involvement leads to loss of objectivity and ability to help. Fostering open communication between child, family and staff goes a long way towards ensuring that a delicate balance is preserved and promotes feelings of mutual care and support.

In children's units safety is a major concern, particularly when dangerous equipment, drugs and solutions are so readily available. Most units now have a written 'safety policy', which should be made available to you, and any questions can be referred to the trained nurses with whom the ultimate responsibility lies.

Whether caring for the child in hospital or at home, many nurses practise 'family centred care' (described below), where the emphasis is very much on the parents as primary care givers, in partnership with nursing and medical staff. When parents are actively involved in caring for their child, problems can arise if they are seen to be demanding or critical of our delivery of care. This is usually a response to the stress and anxiety created by their child's illness and should not be taken personally. It is often helpful to talk such problems through with the sister or charge nurse, so that the situation may be resolved.

Through personal experience as parents, it is tempting to assume that other people's children will behave as yours did at a particular age. However, every child is unique, with different life experiences, personality and cultural background. We must, therefore, strive to find what is right for each and every child in our care, with due regard to their individuality.

Family centred care

The effects of illness and hospitalisation on the child are discussed in detail in the previous section of this chapter. It is therefore the aim of this section to explain to you, the care assistant, how to minimise the harmful effects of illness and hospitalisation on the child, by using a family centred approach when caring for the ill child.

The primary aim of family centred care is to reinforce the parents' ability to care for their child. It takes into account the developmental needs of the child.

By definition, family centred care can not be undertaken without the primary involvement of the family, chiefly the parents. You will recall, developmentally, the child's deep need for his parents; this need is greatly increased during illness. No matter how trivial we may think the child's illness is, his or her parents will be experiencing a degree of guilt in failing to protect their child from trauma, or delaying to seek professional advice. They often worry about their ability to cope and can develop fears of phobic proportions if the child is seriously ill.

Before parents can be involved in the care of their ill child, they must first be understood and supported themselves. They need time to gain confidence in the people who are proposing to take responsibility for their child. The initial contact that the parents have with the carers is of utmost importance in establishing the 'working relationship'. Roles must be defined: the parents are undoubted experts in the needs of their child; the nurse is trained in the care of ill children. The carer should assist the parents in being supportive to their child; without help some parents may make mistakes and feel out of place. If no one takes responsibility for parents it may result in missed opportunities to gain the most from parental presence. Remember that most parents want only what is best for their child. They usually appreciate and accept any reasoning they can understand and are only too eager to share their knowledge in order to obtain the best possible care for their child.

Although the planning of family centred care is not your responsibility, it is important that you understand the process of planning. Family centred care is a collective responsibility. The child, his parents and the nurse are equally involved.

Ultimately, the aim of family centred care is to maintain the normal process of development. If the challenge of childhood illness is to be met and overcome, equal yet different contribution will be required from the child, parents, and the nurse. Together they are equal to the challenge and the outcome can be a rewarding experience.

16

Caring for someone with mental disorder

In this chapter basic ideas about mental disorder will be examined. Questions such as the following will be discussed: what is mental health and disorder? What are the needs of people suffering in this way? What services are available for care and treatment of the individual and support of the family? Who can best help in times of crisis or during more prolonged periods of mental disorder?

The work of the specific members of the mental health care team will be briefly examined and, finally, the help which the carer can give a person in hospital or at home will be considered.

What is mental health and disorder?

There are certain qualities or characteristics which a mentally healthy person possesses. These qualities or abilities enable people to cope effectively with everyday life. The following capacities are shared by all mentally healthy people:

- A realistic awareness of self (strengths, weaknesses, values, attitudes, prejudices, effects of self on others).
- A degree of self-esteem (a valuing of and liking for self).
- An appropriate self-control of feelings or impulses (self-control in both expressing and suppressing important emotions and urges).
- Realistic self-confidence and self-reliance.
- Involvment in personal goals, hobbies, interests at work and home.

- Self-acceptance (warts and all) with a tolerance for own imperfections—no excess of self-criticism.
- A clear perception of reality (the world and other people as they are).
- Enjoyment of persisting and satisfying relationships with others.
- An awareness of and concern (respect) for others.
- An ability to adapt to and cope with life crises.

There is of course, a close relationship between physical and mental health. You have possibly noticed how physical problems can give rise to mental or emotional changes. Someone experiencing breathing difficulties may become temporarily confused and frightened for example. Insufficient or poor diet or dehydration may cause mental deterioration. Toxins from infections (particularly in a child or elderly person) or drugs or alcohol can give rise to an acute delirium. Intense or prolonged emotional stress can also cause physical disorder. Peptic ulcers, high blood pressure, certain skin disorders or asthmatic attacks are examples of these. In a very real sense, then, physical and mental health are intimately linked, and the carer will consider the person as a whole in whatever he or she is doing to help.

There are, nevertheless, a number of people whose health problems are predominantly mental or emotional in nature. Some of these will be less familiar to carers. This relative ignorance of mental disorder can cause anxiety—even fear—in the carer. Lack of understanding about such disorder will also make it difficult to decide how the carer can best help.

Case histories

Mental health is something most of us take for granted. It may not be until something tragic happens (such as attempted suicide or a mother's harm of her young baby) that we become aware that an individual is suffering at all. Consider the following examples of people experiencing mental disorder.

Mrs Jane Manning is 35 years old and married. For most of her married life she has had a morbid fear of travelling in buses, trains or cars. As soon as she thinks about getting into one of these vehicles she becomes anxious, uneasy, restless and panicky.

Eric Johnson is a 19 year old motor mechanic. He is aware of people looking at him. Their eyes are everywhere. They are whispering about him, laughing at him, pointing him out in a crowd. Everywhere the same people are grinning, mocking, taunting.

Jean Rowlands is 48 years old and unmarried. She has slowed up recently and cannot sleep; she is unusually irritable, listless and apathetic. She is no longer interested in her appearance or personal hygiene. She feels an indefinable deep sense of shame. At the same time she has a growing conviction that she is developing a terrible and incurable disease, that she has cancer of the womb.

Mr Thomas Ellis is 69 years old and a widower. He is worried that people are stealing his things. He has so many things to remember lately. He wonders anxiously why his wife isn't home yet? And where has his daughter gone? She lived four doors away only yesterday and yet the people who came to the door swear they have never heard of her! There is something about his daughter, some detail in the back of his mind. If only he could remember.

Mr Stewart Rhodes is a respected local councillor and an elder of the church. He is a Personnel Officer for the local supermarket. He has almost uncontrollable urges to shout obscenities at young women. He avoids contact with them—crosses the road and hides from close female friends. He cloisters himself in the house after work. What kind of beast is he becoming, he wonders?

Consequences of mental disorder may be as follows: total withdrawal of a person from others and everyday life; serious self-neglect, due to profound depression or confusion; social isolation due to morbid fear of going out of the house; total self-starvation due to an obsession with dieting, or increasing dependency upon drugs or alcohol, as attempts to try to deal with excessive stress and anxiety. Clearly, although such people may be physically quite healthy, serious problems have arisen. Their inability to cope fully with life in all its aspects may be total. In addition, the life of a sufferer's family and others can be affected. Parents or children, husband or wife may themselves become unable to cope and friends or workmates experience great difficulty coming to terms with these worrying changes in someone's behaviour.

Unlike a mentally handicapped person, someone with mental disorder has been normal in intellectual and other aspects of development. It is the purpose of the mental health team, with the aid of care and treatment facilities (mental health services), to help such a person return to normality and happiness again.

What are the needs of people suffering mental disorder

Perhaps the first requirement is recognition that mental disorder is present and the second that help and treatment are obtained. People suffering this type of disorder may be unwilling to seek help, due to fear of treatment or of being locked up in a psychiatric hospital. The shame of having to admit mental distress may also prevent early advice and help being sought by sufferer or carer/family member.

Other needs are assessment of the sufferer's behaviour and problems, as well as help for the family who, as already described, may be at their wits end as a result of mental disorder, or in serious financial or domestic difficulties because of temporary loss of parent, husband or wife.

For the few people with mental disorder who may have been in hospital for an extended period, social rehabilitation may be necessary and, depending upon the length of stay in hospital, help with re-employment may be a priority.

Accommodation is sometimes difficult for the mentally disordered person who is recovering from an acute or more chronic stress reaction. Some landlords or families are either unable or unwilling to take the risk of such a person returning to their home, despite reassurance from the psychiatric or social services.

Prevention of further relapse is the last but not least of challenges which the person who has recovered, their family friends and workmates have to face.

What services are available?

Contrary to popular belief, most psychiatric care and treatment is now taking place within the community or on an out-patient or day-patient basis. The number of beds in larger psychiatric hospitals in England have been steadily reducing since the mid 1960s. In fact there was only one hospital with over 1500 beds in the country in 1980. Most psychiatric hospitals contain less than 250 beds (100 in 1976) and an increasing number of patients with mental disorder are treated within small psychiatric units based within a district general hospital (157 such units existed in 1980). Hospital stay is predominantly for short periods only (six to eight weeks approximately) and there are now very few locked wards in psychiatric hospitals. Most patients are able to return home for day visits or weekend leave, during in-patient treatment.

There is an increasing growth in community based care and support facilities. Day-patient attendances have grown from 1740 000 in 1970 to 3423 000 in 1982 and group and hostel places for discharged patients have increased from 3000 to 4000 between 1977 and 1981, although it is recognised that many more places will be needed to meet the demand of increasing numbers of longer stay patients who are returning to the community.

Specialist in-patient and community based facilities are available to meet the needs of the following groups of people with mental disorder: children and adolescents (most work on a five day week basis); alcoholics (both detoxification and rehabilitation units); the more disturbed person (in regional secure units); people who have committed criminal acts as a result of mental disorder (in forensic psychiatric units). In addition, there are in-patient facilities for mothers and their babies following psychiatric disorder after childbirth.

Government training and skill centres, based within the local authority also offer places to people with psychiatric problems from hospital and community with employment difficulties.

Who can help?

The primary health care team and the psychiatric team

The primary health care team (GP, health visitor, district nurse and midwife) work closely with the psychiatric team to provide a comprehensive service. Key members of the psychiatric team include the consultant psychiatrist, mental health nurse, social worker (hospital or community based), psychologist, occupational therapist and resettlement officer.

The consultant psychiatrist and registrar's main responsibilities are to advise on the diagnosis and prescribe treatment for a person suffering some form of mental disorder.

The mental health nurse is responsible for assessing the needs of the sufferer and devising a care approach to help meet these. This may include a range of individual and group psychotherapeutic interventions, such as counselling, goal planning, anxiety management, social skills training or role play. The nurse works closely with the psychiatrist in seeing that prescribed treatments are administered. She also monitors effects of such treatments, reporting regularly to the psychiatrist on progress towards recovery.

The social worker is more concerned with the economic, home and family situation of a person. Developmental and emotional effects on parents, children, husband or wife of a patient can be severe. There may be bills to be paid, others to care for in the home and a variety of domestic or interpersonal problems that need resolving as a result of hospitalisation. It will also be the social worker's responsibility, following requests from relatives or GP, to arrange compulsory admission to hospital for persons suffering acute psychiatric disorder (Mental Health Act 1983).

The psychologist may assist in assessing a person's behaviour or in planning a programme of treatment. He or she may advise on educational developmental matters, particularly in the case of a child or adolescent.

The occupational therapist works closely with others in the team in helping a sufferer regain self-confidence or skills in home management, self-care, or social competency. He or she may be involved in stimulating a person's interest or self-expression by various recreational and craft-based activities.

Each member of the team tries to work closely with the person and family and each other. Often specific professional boundaries are crossed in the interests of continuity of care or treatment. Increasingly, members of the team are working in community based units or even in a person's own home.

The resettlement officer assesses the work skills and potential of a person who has suffered psychiatric disorder and helps reestablish the person in employment.

There are many helpful voluntary local and national groups with special interest in people with mental disorders and their families. One of these is the National Schizophrenia Fellowship (address on page 180). The National Association for Mental Health (MIND) is another active support agency that gives advice on mental health problems, funds research and monitors issues related to mental disorders, including patients' rights. MIND has branches in all cities in the country and the advice centres are open daily.

The role of the care assistant

The general role of the carer will be to support the person suffering mental disorder and the family members. He or she will work closely with others (members of both the primary and psychiatric team) to help in restoration and maintenance of mental health. This may involve helping someone with activities of daily living, such as eating, dressing, attending to their personal hygiene and other aspects of self-care. Each of these everyday personal tasks may become a problem for someone because of severe depression or confusion. Excess anxiety or preoccupation with delusional ideas or hallucinations can also be distressing and carers will need to assist in determining the presence and severity of these problems, as well as in protecting the sufferer and others from harm due to suicidal or aggressive impulses precipitated by mental distress.

Even the most severe form of mental disorder will eventually respond to modern treatment. One important contribution the carer can make is to instil hope in this eventual recovery, thereby combating a sense of hopelessness, anguish or despair felt by a mentally disordered person.

Some common problems

Some guidance on how the carer can help in more specific problem situations may now be useful. It is beyond the scope of this chapter, however, to go beyond more than basic principles in assisting a mentally disordered person. What follows, therefore, are suggestions to help a person during different phases of mental disorder. The more common difficulties related to mental disorder are severe depression, excessive anxiety, suicidal or aggressive impulses, distress caused by hallucinations (voices are more common than other sensory abnormalities), delusional ideas and severe confusion and delirium.

A preliminary to all helping approaches is for the carer to establish and maintain an effective relationship with the person experiencing mental disorder. Key qualities the carer needs to consider in the relationship are acceptance of the person without direct criticism or patronising attitudes. A genuine concern needs to be transmitted and respect and empathy shown. Common courtesies and sensitivity to the sufferer's feelings are of course important, as well as honesty and mutual trust. Establishing such a relationship may take time and needs to proceed at the pace indicated by the disturbed person.

Anxiety

Someone undergoing an acute anxiety reaction—perhaps a panic attack—can be helped in the following way. The carer approaches the panicky person in a calm, slow way, perhaps offering reassuring hand pressure or embrace. The carer should speak in a calm, clear voice, perhaps slightly slower and lower in tone than normal. It is often useful if the person can be gently persuaded to sit down, as they may be feeling particularly physically distressed at this time, even faint and breathless. As soon as the person is a little more composed—and this stage should not be rushed—the reasons for the panic state should be explored. If these are due to misunderstanding or lack of knowledge then clear explanation or information should be offered by the carer if this is available. When the cause of the panic is worry about some real or imagined event, the person could be helped to take some positive action to resolve this. This often restores the person's confidence and faith in him/herself and others.

In some instances helping the person to de-escalate their increasing anxiety by encouraging physical relaxation, particularly by lying down, and taking deep, slow breaths will help. These are specific techniques of self-relaxation which the person can easily learn using audio tapes and simple step by step instructions. These exercises are particularly useful when there seem to be no clear triggers to the panic attack or excess anxiety.

Depression

Sometimes a person may be severely depressed and withdrawn. Talking quietly with such a person may be very comforting, or not talking at all but staying close beside the person in their despair. If the depressed person feels like crying or becoming angry, then let them feel that it is acceptable to let these feelings out. Considerable relief may be obtained after a good cry, particularly if the person feels that the carer is not embarrassed by such tears or frustration. It may be helpful for the very sad person to talk about happier times they have experienced, or to be reassured firmly that they will surely come through this miserable phase. Again, hand holding and other physical contact, if acceptable, can be most consoling. It is important to realise that as a carer in this situation, you may feel quite exhausted after a while. So do share the responsibility of supporting the depressed person with others.

Aggression

Occasionally someone suffering mental disorder may become verbally or physically aggressive. This can be quite a frightening experience for a carer and a general principle is not to try to cope with such a person alone. At least one other person should be involved, as there is less risk of harm due to your own panic or over-reaction, or the excess activity of the sufferer. It is helpful if you can maintain a confident, poised, calm, unhurried approach and exterior at this time. This may not be easy but comes with practice. If your own anxiety, panic or anger is perceived, then these reactions may amplify the person's own hostility or fear. (Fear is often a cause of hostility.) The frustrated or angry person may need more personal space and an opportunity to ventilate such feelings, by throwing or banging things or hitting inanimate objects. Considerable relief is often obtained following this. It is useful to remember that damage to objects or property is much less harmful than damage to self or others. In the event of an actual physical attack, the key thing to bear in mind is restraint, rather than retaliation. Where possible, holding the person's wrists or pinning arms to sides might help. The safest position for the carer is behind the aggressive person and ideally both attacker and carer should be on the floor, where there is far less risk of harm to either. Removal of shoes is a wise precaution. Sufficient restraint should be applied to the arms, legs and head, where possible, to prevent blows. This is best done by firmly holding the joints at the elbows, knees, shoulders or ankles. On no account should a person be restrained by the neck. It is also risky if pressure is put on the abdomen, particularly if the aggressive person is pregnant!

It is a matter of good judgement as to when restraint should be released. Talking to the aggressive person throughout, helping him to realise that no harm is intended by those restraining, is often reassuring. When control is released, the carer should try to reassure the person of her continuing concern and support, despite this often traumatic episode.

A careful analysis of the situation—possible causes of the aggression and evaluation of the action taken—should be undertaken. Lastly, any injury sustained by anyone should be assessed, treated, reported and carefully recorded.

Hallucinations and delusions

Some forms of mental disorder cause a person to become very suspicious of others, particularly a close friend or significant family members. Behind this kind of reaction may be influences of persecutory voices—as a form of hallucination. At the same time the sufferer's thoughts can become unusual or strange. Odd beliefs may be expressed—that peculiar things are happening around him, or that there is imminent danger from others close by. This person may consequently become quite afraid and withdrawn or become unable to express ideas or feelings clearly. Total isolation from everyone may be the result of such an experience.

The carer will need to adopt a patient and non-intrusive, non-threatening approach at this time. He or she must try to build up slowly but steadily the person's trust in him or her. It can be difficult for someone who is suspicious and thus too frightened to tolerate company at first, when the mere presence of the carer and others seem threatening. Usually short but relatively frequent periods of contact are best and the fewer people involved at this time the better. The carer will need to demonstrate that he or she can be relied upon and be consistent in day to day contact. Any promises made must be kept. Nothing should be done to increase feelings of suspicion: no whispering, laughing in corners or pointing at the person, for example. An open, honest, frank attitude is essential. It is a good policy to explain any actions, procedures or treatments very clearly and carefully to allay any doubts or anxieties. Sometimes food or prescribed medication may be rejected, in the belief that these are poisoned. The person should not be forced to eat or take prescribed tablets. Gentle persuasion and calm persistence will usually work, particularly as the person's trust is won. Food may be accepted from a trusted friend or relative, or the person may feel safer eating food he has prepared himself or got from a tin or packet, which he has opened.

Bringing the person into any conversation, particularly with family or friends, about him will reduce misunderstanding and worry. On the other hand, the suspicious person's need to be alone and private should be respected. Group activities or pressure to join in things may increase defensiveness.

Suspicious people usually feel better if they have some control over events. This can be achieved by involvement in decision about how their day is organised, establishing simple rules, determining likes, dislikes and interests and respecting choices or wishes wherever possible.

At night, sleep may be especially troublesome and the person may be afraid to close his or her eyes for fear of harm. A low light in the bedroom, or the presence of a trusted person in the room may allay such anxiety and fear and promote sleep.

If hallucinatory voices are distressing then conversation or simple diversional techniques from the carer may dispel these. The person may find listening to music or other recreational pursuits dispels these distressing voices.

There may be odd ideas or beliefs disclosed to the carer that may be upsetting. It is advisable to accept these without criticism or argument. However, delusional ideas should not be agreed with, but tactfully discontinued as being difficult to accept as true by the carer. It is important to realise though that such beliefs can be very real and strong for the sufferer. Listening carefully and responding more to the feelings behind the person's statements will help increase a sense of acceptance and safety.

Confusion

Mental disorder may present in the form of acute or chronic confusion. Older people and the very young are vulnerable to this, as is anyone abusing alcohol or drugs. Sometimes infections or a sudden change of environment, particularly in an older person, produce confusion.

Extreme restlessness, even exhaustion can result from confusion and great demands will be made upon the skills and resources of the carer at such a time. Considerable patience and reassurance will be needed in the care of a confused person. Slower, simple phrases, often repeated a few times to reinforce meaning, can help.

Careful attention to explaining names and orientating the confused person to daily events and her environment will be necessary. A confused person will have difficulty remembering her way about, her routines, time of day, even recent happenings in her life, or people and places. Large notices, identifying key areas in the home or hospital will be useful. A large calendar and clock can give clues to date and time. Radio and television programmes provide up to date information and interest. An elderly person will feel less alienated if she has personal items around. Photographs or ornaments, for example, on her bedside locker will remind a confused person of familiar people and things.

It is important also to ensure that the older confused person wears her usual hearing aid or glasses, as loss of these increases isolation and frustration.

A fairly structured daily programme of activities give a sense of security and purpose to someone who is muddled. Regular times for meals, personal care, going to the toilet become little landmarks in the day. Enough stimulation to keep the confused person in contact with daily life, but not so much that she becomes overwhelmed, will be invaluable.

A confused person's safety and protection from hazards in their environment will be another part of the carer's responsibility. Hot liquids, slippery floors, gas taps and electric wires are some potential dangers. When someone is confused they are more likely to wander off and get lost. On a cold day or night this could be fatal.

It is easy to take over all self-care of a confused person. There is much satisfaction in helping others and often so little time to spare. If the independence and dignity of an older person is not preserved, then the quality of their daily life is impoverished. The carer then needs to recognise opportunities to reinforce the confused individual's abilities and self-respect and maintain their grasp, however tentative, on reality.

However, it would be equally harmful to over-protect a confused person, limiting activities, outings and independence unnecessarily.

Conclusion

Caring for someone with mental disorder can be interesting, challenging and rewarding. Whether you are based in a hospital or in the community, or a husband, wife, son or daughter of a sufferer, you will find this experience a significant one. Do remember that the experienced professionals are there to help and that modern treatment and facilities for care and rehabilitation are invariably effective. No one need fear mental disorder for everyone can be helped in some way.

17

Working with people with a mental handicap

This chapter will consider ways in which people approach and work with children and adults who have learning difficulties. The term 'mental handicap' in itself is somewhat misleading and many people often associate it with images of deviance and low esteem. For others it conjures up feelings of insecurity, fear and apprehension.

However, there is another group of people who regard people with a mental handicap as being different in other ways from 'normal people' and as such go out of their way to be pleasant, patronising and are over-cautious in providing people with opportunities to take risks or to live like other people for fear of causing unnecessary trauma or anxiety to them.

Perception of mental handicap

The opening sentences of this chapter are deliberately chosen to challenge and to make you consider your own perception of what a person with a mental handicap means to you. Surprisingly many of us come into contact with people with learning difficulties in a wide variety of settings, which are certainly not limited to services provided by statutory agencies, such as the DH and DSS.

People with mental handicaps are people first and, like you or I, have very real and ordinary feelings and experiences which, given the opportunity to emerge and develop, will demand the same skills and approach as we afford to other people who may use our services. It would be wrong to presume that a person with a mental handicap does not have additional needs, but as a starting point to this chapter it is perhaps more appropriate to consider them as individuals with similar needs to ourselves, whilst recognising that they may take a little longer to acquire or consolidate some of the learning experiences that we take for granted in our everyday lives.

There are many myths surrounding the concept of mental handicap, for example the association of mental handicap with violence and crime and the idea that every person with a mental handicap is mentally ill. Research and experience has shown that not only are these associations untrue and unfounded, but that they help people in society to label or conveniently categorise people who do not fit easily into conventional lifestyles that we take for granted to be normal in our own neighbourhood. Essentially the incidence of mental illness, violence or disturbed behaviour is no higher than that of any other person living in the community or in your neighbourhood. Having dispensed with this point, we can now begin to give people with a mental handicap a chance to present themselves as valued, caring and equal members of society, having a right to expect from us the opportunities they require to enjoy a meaningful life without hindrance or unnecessary attention being drawn to themselves.

Case history

In order to discuss this point further, let us illustrate, through the use of a case study, some of the points identified above.

John and Jane Paterson were in their early 20s and were looking forward to their first child. They had secured a comfortable home close to their family and were enjoying the expectations of imminent parenthood. John and Jane were both healthy, with no previous history of mental handicap in either family and like other expectant parents attended antenatal and parentcraft sessions, where they shared their aspirations of future parenthood. Jane gave birth to a strong, bouncy baby boy who was physically well and demanded from his parents the same life as any other child. They called him Stephen.

Stephen had Down's syndrome, which is a congenital condition and the most common of all diagnosed mental handicap syndromes. The joy of parenthood was shattered for Jane and her husband; the diagnosis was made immediately at birth. The paediatrician and midwife offered support and a health visitor offered counselling and promise of follow-up care at home. All these people were total strangers and were hardly a substitute for family and friends, whom Jane looked to for support and encouragement following the birth of her child. Few visited her and they found it difficult to share her reactions.

Stephen grew up to be a happy, healthy young boy and with the help of her family, who soon rallied round, Jane and her husband forged close links in their local neighbourhood and were soon proud to take Stephen out for walks and enjoy integrating him with normal play groups; instead segregating him with other 'handicapped children', Stephen had playmates and friends just like everyone else. Later Jane and her husband were able to say how pleased they were with the help and support they had received from caring professionals and understanding neighbours, but most important they realised they themselves had taken the first steps to ease the difficulties which others faced in sharing Stephen. They had come to terms with his birth and made a concerted decision that from the word go he would not be different from other children, but would hold his head high in the crowd just like any other person.

Stephen went on to attend a normal school and although he did not manage to achieve as well as some other children, with some prompting and support he managed to spend his school days in a peer group of children without learning difficulties and have a start in life to benefit from the same advantages and opportunities as his friends.

Readers may be surprised to hear how positive this story is but it is not uncommon for such stories to be shared. Not all children with learning difficulties would be as fortunate as Stephen, in being able to cultivate and develop their own learning to a level which enables them to share with other children in ordinary learning environments. However, the same principles apply in that if a child such as Stephen is treated as normally as possible and not sheltered and protected from the same challenges and rules of life, there is the same chance of him developing to his maximum potential and meeting the expectations of society afforded to other children.

Where, then, do professionals come in to enable this process to unfold? Unquestionably, the first approach is one of attitude. We ourselves must come to terms with the fact that children with learning difficulties are, in fact, no different from other children; by showing this, we will help parents to understand that we have every intention of providing them with the support that they so need. We must, in effect, take Jane and John back to the days prior to Stephen's birth and help to realise some of the expectations they had of having a healthy child. Let us list some of those expectations:

- The birth of a child who will contribute to the family and bring love and warmth and pride
- A child who will attract interest, companionship and recognition from neighbours and family
- Somebody with whom the family can share their love, resources and home.

These are but a few of the expectations that parents have of a new-born child and in all of these a person with a mental handicap can offer many of the rewards of parenthood. What is different is that the family will take longer to adjust to the birth of their child and have to learn new coping strategies which may be unfamiliar to their own parents and to local neighbours. The parents will, therefore, need to provide new learning opportunities for other members of their family to ensure that their new child is fully integrated and welcomed to the family.

Professionals and carers will often be in touch with families and children with learning difficulties and the way in which parents perceive others' reactions to their child will be of paramount importance in helping them to develop their own coping strategies of coming to terms with their child. In particular, the most familiar person to get to know the parents will be the nursing auxiliary or care assistant in the maternity unit and subsequently in out-patient departments and during episodes of acute admission.

Unfortunately, some children with mental handicaps have associated physical disorders, such as those connected with spasticity, cardiac insufficiency and epilepsy. During childhood a large number of these children will undergo extensive diagnostic tests and treatment which will often require their admission to hospital. It is during these episodes that parents will meet professionals for the first time and have to learn how to share in the care of their children. Most of these admissions take place in the early years of life before the child has had a chance to attend school. Parents are still suspicious and somewhat concerned in respect of their own capability of working with their children and are particularly anxious about sharing their 'special child' with others.

So far this chapter has helped us to focus on our own perceptions of mental handicap and this will be put to the test in how we meet and approach the children when they come to us for care. What is important to note is that people with mental handicaps may not be in a position to have developed the same level of verbal response and comprehension we expect of normal children. Children with brain damage may take longer to acquire the basic use of language and understanding. In a world devoid of full comprehension, a child with learning difficulties may become suspicious, concerned and frightened by unfamiliar noises and people.

Admission to hospital

The best of us find it difficult to adapt to change and this is particularly true when we are not in control of the situation. Hence admission to hospital for any child is a time of intense insecurity and concern, but for a child with learning difficulties, who may be used to a simple routine that he/she has learned during the early years of life, it is particularly hard to adapt to strange voices, glaring lights and new smells, etc.

Although the command of language may be delayed in some children, there is no reason to suggest that their other senses are undeveloped. In fact, on the contrary, many children are hypersensitive to touch, light, temperature and sudden noises. What is required is an approach which encourages gentle stimulation of all senses, which will reassure the child and provide an opportunity for the messages we are trying to impart to be delivered in a way the child understands.

The first thing to consider is to reassure parents by sitting down and discussing the child's likes and dislikes and, in particular, be sure to ask the ways in which the child communicates his/her basic needs. The child, for example, may have a particular way of gesturing or a particular intonation to ask to use the toilet or reject a particular food. Nurses working with people with a mental handicap on a full-time basis are fully aware of the need to take a detailed history of such events and interests. Similarly, it is essential to discover what the child finds particularly distressing or dislikes, since this will only encourage withdrawal into an alien world or cause the child to react through insecurity and demonstrate behaviour that some nurses and care staff find it difficult to cope with.

It is also important to share with parents every aspect of treatment and diagnosis, since this may be the first time they have been separated from their child. This, of course, is not unfamiliar when working in paediatric wards with children without learning difficulties, but it is important to note that many parents believe there is no other person able to understand their child, since they have particular needs and communications systems which parents have often had to keep to themselves. Sensitivity in understanding these basic needs is required to provide the parents and child with an opportunity to enjoy and make the most of the admission.

As described above, some children will have clinical needs which require additional attention. Epilepsy is one such condition, which is present in some 25% of children with severe learning difficulties and may be a direct result of brain damage. Parents often feel particularly anxious with epilepsy but careful and controlled understanding of the condition and a response from nurses and care staff, which is both rehearsed and confident, will help parents to allay many of their fears.

Although it used to be that many children with mental handicap died early, nowadays many survive into adult life or old age. The principles of care for these people should ensure that they are cared for safely, allowed individual choices in life, enjoy as normal a life as possible and receive all necessary social and health care. Parents and relatives need help if this is to be achieved. For example, if a care worker over-reacts to a simple situation, such as an epileptic seizure, parents will become very anxious. The procedure for handling epileptic seizures is, in fact, very straightforward and simple to handle. However, many care workers find epileptic seizures distressing and staff require preparation and prior knowledge of how to handle such a situation, when it occurs. Basically the procedure is to ensure that the person is removed from any dangerous obstacles or situations. During a typical major epileptic seizure, an individual will lose consciousness for between two and four minutes and will fall to the floor and shake vigorously. This can be most distressing to watch, although the individual concerned will usually feel any ill effects after the seizure, which will usually be worked through quite naturally, once the shaking has subsided. If possible, the individual should be laid on his or her side, away from potentially harmful objects, and support be given to the neck to prevent the tongue being swallowed, thus causing asphyxiation. No drinks should be given to the individual and tight clothing should be removed. Should the individual be in danger of falling close to stairs or to a window, then attempts should be made to remove the individual immediately. However, in normal circumstances, it is better to leave the individual where he or she falls to allow him or her to work through the seizure. During the recovery phase, the person may feel confused and bewildered. It is important to re-orientate the person by sitting with him or her and helping the adjustment to reality as he or she recovers.

There are very few clinical conditions associated with mental handicap that require special treatment. However, there are a number of people with a mental handicap who will have associated sensory deficits as well. In this book you will find reference to working with children and adults who have both visual and hearing defects; people with a mental handicap may also have these additional difficulties to cope with.

Rubella is a condition which combines both physical and

mental handicaps with blindness or deafness. Rubella is associated with German measles, which is contracted during the
early stages of pregnancy and may result in the production of a
multiple handicap. Those who were infected by the rubella virus
require particular help and understanding, since they have
sensory deficits and will often be isolated within a world which
offers little stimulation. A multidisciplinary approach to care is
required, which will often need the expertise of many therapists
at one time or another. Physiotherapists, speech therapists,
occupational therapists, psychologists and care staff will all be
involved in developing appropriate treatment, which care assistants will be asked to implement. These may range from simple
feeding programmes to helping the individual to learn a manual
signing system to indicate their needs when they are unable to
verbalise their requests. Some may feel the world offers little
opportunities to such individuals, but evidence has shown that
when concerted efforts are made to provide additional stimulation for such people they are in fact able to acquire new skills and
develop to a level whereby they can understand and contribute
to an active life at home and in the community.

It is particularly important to seek advice from physiotherapists in respect of providing appropriate seating and
mobility aids for those who have additional multiple handicaps,
such as the ones associated with cerebral palsy. Cerebral palsy,
or spasticity, as it is more commonly known, may also be associated with brain damage. However, this is not always the case
and in some situations it is difficult to assess the level of brain
damage involved. It is therefore essential to remember that such
children and adults may have a highly developed level of comprehension which should never be taken for granted. This illustrates the most important rule for care staff to remember, that
although a person with a mental handicap or spasticity may
appear not to comprehend what is happening around them, it is
always essential to value and to respect the person's privacy and
treat him or her as if he or she is fully conversant with you. It is so
easy to talk around him or her to other members of staff or to
address the individual in a patronising or simple fashion,
without giving credit for the individual's level of understanding.
One of the ground rules is therefore to respect the individual's

dignity—always address the person by name and never dis-
regard a person's level of awareness.

Spasticity presents particular problems when associated with
a mental handicap. Learning in itself is a difficult experience,
which requires opportunities to explore the world in order to
learn and assimilate many of the things we take for granted. A
person who is mentally handicapped and has limited mobility
has particular difficulty in conquering and experiencing his
everyday environment. Care staff will need to be particularly
aware that additional opportunities must be provided to stimulate children, who are often confined to wheelchairs and may
find their world very limited in scope and experience.

Teaching such children and adults to acquire new skills and to
develop to their maximum potential requires particular
ingenuity and understanding of their needs. However, care staff
will often be most directly involved in providing opportunities to
create meaningful learning environments. Attention should be
given to the routine offered to a child or adult in such circumstances. Variation of routine, re-positioning, a change of chair
during the day and a change of scenery are all basic, but an
important part of enriching the quality of life. A change of scene,
such as being taken out of the ward for a while and given some
one to one attention, will always help to stimulate a person's
learning ability.

In some hospitals toy libraries are provided, where expert
advice may be sought from trained toy librarians and therapists
on the most appropriate toys to choose to stimulate learning,
when a particular stage of learning has been identified. Play is a
therapeutic medium for children and adults with learning difficulties, since it is, after all, our first introduction to the world:
through trial and error learning and experience, we learn to make
sense of basic shapes, objects and how they relate to us. Also
important is an understanding of one's own body image and it is
helpful to draw the attention of an adult or a child to their own
profile in a mirror through the introduction of games that identify the person's body image.

Most important, it is essential to remember that each child or
adult is an individual with different needs and different
experiences; it would be wrong to assume that there is one simple

strategy to help any one person with a mental handicap. In order to develop this individuality and to help the person to feel valued, it is essential to get to know him or her. Assessment is a key tool to understanding the needs of individuals and, rather than talk about the things they cannot do, it is more useful and practical to talk about the things they can do and thereafter identify ways of building on existing skills to make them more independent.

Not so many years ago, people with mental handicaps were labelled and identified by a measure of their intelligence quotient or IQ. I am sure that if somebody told you that a person had an IQ of 56 it would have little meaning to you, apart from telling you that he or she was not as bright as a normal person. This particular measure tells us little about a person's abilities and is quite useless when translated into attempts to help people to develop or to understand their needs.

The use of assessment procedures to see how well someone is performing in areas such as dressing, feeding, walking, talking or continence are all more meaningful descriptions, which will help to contribute to develop skills for everyday life. Therefore assessments tend to be made about daily living skills and a person's particular level of performance at any given time. Once we have identified the level of function, it is often possible to develop exercises and programmes to help teach individuals to progress to the next stage of learning in that particular area. The same applies to our own childhood experiences as we learn to talk or to count or to dress ourselves. People with a mental handicap may take a little longer but need as much positive encouragement and stimulation as we had when we were young to develop to a level which they can justifiably feel proud of. Time and patience is required when teaching people with a mental handicap, for rewards and progress may be slow. However, experiences show many care workers that perseverance and understanding will be justly rewarded when small but significant strides are made towards independence.

We have already said in this chapter that people with a mental handicap find change difficult to accept and sometimes too many changes in the environment may cause levels of anxiety and stress which cannot always be understood. An inability to understand feelings or to describe or discuss how one feels may result in alternative methods of demonstrating concern or anxiety. Occasionally, behaviour problems may occur that may be associated with a means of telling us that the individual feels unhappy or confused. Changes in staff are not uncommon in paediatric wards or in mental handicap units and yet we so often take for granted the impact that the loss of a close care worker may have on an individual. Hence it is not surprising that the sudden loss of a caring friend or a change of ward or routine or temporary absence of parents may cause insecurity. It is not unusual for individuals to react to such situations by becoming distressed, tearful or angry. People with a mental handicap are not usually violent and indeed in most situations where this occurs the reason, if sought, is usually linked to a sudden change in a person's routine or a failure of care staff to understand a person's needs. We need to be particularly careful in interpreting such needs, since many people with mental handicaps are unable to provide us with the answers. Observation skills, listening skills and common sense will often be the tools in use, noticing the subtle changes in a person's behaviour which may lead us to understand that he or she is distressed or uncomfortable. By knowing the children or adults personally one can often avert potential disturbances which have so often damaged the image of people with a mental handicap.

Conclusion

This chapter has looked at ways in which we treat our work with children and adults who have learning difficulties. The chapter started by appraising the way in which we view and treat people with learning difficulties and to assess how we help them to become contributing individuals in society. People with mental handicaps have the same basic rights as any other person and should be afforded opportunities to develop and realise those rights. This is really a basic, fundamental principle in trying to make their lives 'as normal as possible', whilst remembering that special needs will also need to be met. It is important to remember that people with a mental handicap have a right to:

- Be loved and to share in everyday experiences in life
- The opportunity to leave home and seek an alternative valued home of choice
- The opportunity to seek valued and meaningful employment
- Choose and make friends and have interpersonal experiences like anyone else
- Say 'no' and a right to have a choice in what is happening to them, rather than to sit back as passive recipients of services
- A variety of opportunities and friends to make their lives more meaningful
- Receive adequate finance from the DSS to live as independently as possible within their own means without expecting charity from society.

Children with mental handicaps grow up to become adults and one hopes that during the formative years of childhood many of the obvious handicaps that they were born with will have been overcome by positive learning experiences in their environment. The most important test of success will be linked to the number of friends and positive successes the individual has achieved during life. The way in which we react to people with mental handicaps is therefore a central determinant of the success or failure that such people will have on us as members of society. We need to change our attitude to ensure that we provide new experiences and opportunities and remember that each person is an individual in his or her own right. Allowing time, patience, friendship and experiences can provide us all with many opportunities to share what society has to offer.

18

Where next?

Most people who work as care assistants consider the value of further education and training. All sorts of opportunities present themselves from evening classes to professional courses in universities, colleges or schools of nursing. Many local colleges run part-time afternoon and evening classes for carers. These may be based on specific course outlines, such as those developed by the Open University, or may arise due to local demand. An example of such a course is a 'back to nursing' course in association with a local hospital or a short evening class programme on communicating with the deaf person, put on at the request of the RNID. The Open University courses are especially attractive and valuable programmes with titles such as 'Caring for Older People' (P650), 'Mental Handicap: Patterns for Living (P555) and 'Rehabilitation: A Collaborative Approach to Work with Disabled People' (P556). It is always worthwhile checking if these are available at your local college before writing to the Open University, Walton Hall, Milton Keynes MK7 6AA, for their information package. There are alternative 'open' or 'distance learning' courses available at many colleges. These can be courses preparing you for GCSE examination or be appropriate for self-learning in a special subject that interests you. An example of such a programme is 'Caring for Patients with Cancer' which is published by the Distance Learning Centre for Nursing based at Barnet College, London, and Central Manchester College.

Training to be a nurse is an attractive proposition for many people who enjoy caring or working as hospital volunteers.

Nurses, contrary to popular newspapers are not all blond, shapely, eighteen year old females. They come in all shapes, sizes, ages and sexes, and they work in a wide variety of nursing settings. If you are seriously interested in nursing training you can obtain information from several sources. It is probably easiest to go along to your local library or job centre and ask about local opportunities. Currently three year training pro-grammes are available for general nursing (RGN), mental handi-cap nursing (RNMH) and mental illness nursing (RMN). One can qualify as a sick children's nurse (RSCN), a community nurse (DN, CPN or HV) or a midwife (RM) only as a second qualifica-tion, although this will change as the plans for changing nursing education, are implemented. You will find most courses involve full-time commitment (37½ hours per week) but part-time courses are increasing in number and it is always worthwhile enquiring. Once you know what is available write or telephone for an appointment to discuss nurse training at the hospital. Ask to speak to the director of nurse education, since he or she is the best person to advise. Before keeping your appointment it is wise to find out more of what nursing involves. The DH provides free leaflets on request from DH Leaflet Office, PO Box 21, Stan-more, Middlesex HA7 1AY. You should ask for the general leaf-let 'Nursing' and any specific leaflets relating to your area of interest.

To find out about course admission procedure, type of pro-grammes offered and the variety of courses available, you should consult the Nurses Central Clearing House (NCCH) handbook. This is often available in libraries or Job Centres or can be obtained by post from ENB NCCH, PO BOX 346, Bristol BS99 7FB (telephone 0272 292282). A small fee is charged for the handbook. Both the DH and NCCH give addresses for training institutes outside England.

There are many other posts in hospitals and in the community which do not require such intensive preparation or the irregular hours that nursing involves. Most hospitals, health authorities and social service departments have vacancies from time to time for care assistants, auxiliary staff and home helps. These are usually advertised in the local press or job centre but you can always express your interest in writing, asking to be considered when a vacancy arises. When discussing the post always ask about training and ensure that the employer, if a private agency, is offering the nationally agreed wage. Job centres have details of these rates.

Other specialised courses available at local colleges provide instruction for nursery nurses, dental nurses, chiropody assistants, child minders or play therapists. Although some of these have been seen as courses for school leavers, others are especially for the older applicant. Some colleges offer special courses in health care for those who wish to become care assistants.

The other major caring profession is, of course, social work. Social workers' qualifications can be obtained through degree or diploma studies, with special schemes for older candidates available in many areas of the country. These are especially attractive to those mature applicants who have few formal examination qualifications, but have experience, aptitude, intelligence and motivation. Qualified social workers are employed in hospital and in the community working in wide areas of care from child abuse to the probation services. Opportunity is available for specialisation. Many centres welcome the older applicant with family commitments and, as with nursing, financial aid is available during training. Further information is available from the Central Council for Education and Training in Social Work (CCETSW) offices at the following addresses:

- Derbyshire House, St Chad's Street, London WC1H 8AD
- 9 South St David Street, Edinburgh EH2 2BW
- West Wing, St David's House, Wood Street, Cardiff CF1 1ES
- 14 Malone Road, Belfast BT9 5BN
- Your local college or social work department.

As with nursing, course recruitment is centralised and leaflets from these enquiry offices give all necessary information relating to all courses. Many courses can be studied part-time, some include work experience and others can be undertaken whilst working as an unqualified social worker.

Perhaps, though, you do not feel able to take on a job or a course of study. You can always join local college classes without formal examination or assessment and, if you have others who are interested in learning about certain subjects, you can always approach the head of caring courses about providing a course for you. There are many opportunities for voluntary workers and these posts can give you insight into the various options available. Do not forget to use your local library and, if you are working in a hospital or in the community, check if they have access to a library that you can use. Some journals readily available on book stalls may interest you and, if you ask at your local library you may find local groups which you can join. The addresses on pages 178–181 will be useful if you wish to join local groups who share similar interests.

All in all, the answer to 'Where next is really up to you. It is difficult to make decisions immediately about your future but there are many people and plenty of information available to help you decide. Do not be afraid to seek guidance and advice on such an important decision. After all, carers are very important people and making the right choice is important not only to you but to those you care for. An unhappy carer is not much good to anyone!

Further reading

BRAIN J and MARTIN M D (1980)
Child Care and Health for Nursery Nurses. Hulton Education
Publications Limited, Cheltenham.

DHSS leaflet D49 (1987)
What to do after a death. DHSS, London.

FLACK M and JOHNSTON M (1986)
Handbook for Care. Beaconsfield, Beaconsfield, Eng.

GRAY M and McKENZIE H (1980)
Take Care of your Elderly Relative. Allen and Unwin, and
Beaconsfield, Beaconsfield.

HENDERSON VV (1966)
The Nature of Nursing. MacMillan, London.

MANDELSTAM D (1980)
Incontinence and its Management. Croom Helm, London.

MARTIN JP (1984)
Hospitals in Trouble. Blackwell Scientific Publications, Oxford.

OPEN UNIVERSITY (1986)
Distance Learning Package.
Mental Handicap—Patterns for Living. Open University,
Milton Keynes.

ROPER N, LOGAN W and TIERNEY A (1981)
Learning to use the Process of Nursing. Churchill Livingstone,
Edinburgh.

St John Ambulance Association, St Andrew's Ambulance Association and the British Red Cross Society (1987) First aid manual 5th ed. Dorling, Kindersley, London.

SINES D T and BICHNELL J (1985)
Caring for Mentally Handicapped People in the Community. Harper and Row, London.

WELLER B F (1980)
Helping Sick Children Play. Baillière Tindall, London.

Useful addresses

This is a short list of the most important services referred to in the text. Local offices can be located through the telephone directory or through the reference section in the public library.

Age Concern England (National Old People's Welfare Council)
Bernard Sunley House, 60 Pitcairn Road, Mitcham

The Arthritis and Rheumatism Council for Research
Faraday House, 8/10 Charing Cross Road, London WC2

Asthma Research Council
12 Pembridge Square, London W2 4EH

BACUP
121/123 Charterhouse Street, London EC1M 6AA

British Association for Service to the Elderly
7 Victoria Gardens, Victoria Avenue, Hull

British Diabetic Association
10 Queen Anne Street, London W1M OBD

British Epilepsy Association
New Wokingham Road, Wokingham, Berkshire

British Heart Foundation
57 Gloucester Place, London W1H 4DH

British Homeopathic Association
27a Devonshire Street, London W1N 1RJ

British Library of Tape Recordings for Hospital Patients
12 Lant Street, London SE1 1QR

Cancer Relief
Michael Sobell House, 30 Dorset Square, London NW1 6QL

The Chest, Heart and Stroke Association
Tavistock House North, Tavistock Square, London WC1H 9JE

Colostomy Welfare Group
38–39 Eccleston Square (2nd Floor), London SW1

The Compassionate Friends
5 Lower Clifton Hill Clifton, Bristol

Cripples' Help Society (Manchester, Salford and North West England)
26 Blackfriars Street, Manchester M3 5BE

CRUSE (The National Organisation for the Widowed and their Children)
Cruse House, 126 Sheen Road, Richmond, Surrey TW9 1UR

Disabled Drivers Association
The Hall, Ashwellthorpe, Norwich NR16 1EX

Disabled Living Foundation
346 Kensington High Street, London W14 8NS (Tel: 01 289 6111)

Gingerbread
35 Wellington St, London WC2E 7BN

Ileostomy Association of Great Britain and Northern Ireland
Drove Cottage, Fuzzy Drove, Kempshott, Basingstoke, Hants

Institute of Religion and Medicine
St Margaret's Vicarage, St Margaret's Road, Oxford OX2 6RX

Invalid Childrens Aid Association (London Incorporated)
126 Buckingham Palace Road, London SW1W 9SB

Liverpool Children's Welfare Trust
34 Stanley Street, Liverpool L1 6AN

Marie Curie Memorial Foundation
124 Sloane Street, London SW1X 9BP

MIND (National Association for Mental Health)
22 Harley Street, London W1N 2ED

Multiple Sclerosis Society of Great Britain and Northern Ireland
286 Munster Road, Fulham, London SW6 6AP

National Association for the Welfare of Children in Hospital
Exton House, 7 Exton Street, London SE1 8UE

National Children's Bureau
8 Wakeley Street, London EC1V 7QE

National League for the Blind and Disabled
2 Tenterden Road, Tottenham, London N17 8BE

National Library for the Blind
Cromwell Road, Bredbury, Stockport SK6 2SG

National Schizophrenia Fellowship
78/79 Victoria Road, Surbiton, Surrey KT6 4NS

National Society for Autistic Children
1A Golders Green Road, London NW11 8EA

National Society for Cancer Relief
Michael Sobell House, 30 Dorset Square, London NW1 6QL

National Society for Mentally Handicapped Children and Adults
National Centre, 117/123 Golden Lane, London EC1Y ORT

The Order of St John
St John's Gate, Clerkenwell, London EC1M 4DA

Parkinson's Disease Society
36 Portland Place, London W1N 3DG

The Patients Association
11 Dartmouth Street, London SW1H 9BN

Royal Association in aid of the Deaf and Dumb
7–11 Armstrong Road, Acton, London W3 7JL

The Royal Association for Disability and Rehabilitation
25 Mortimer Street, London W1N 8AB

Royal National Institute for the Blind
224 Great Portland Street, London W1N 6AA

Royal Society of Tropical Medicine and Hygiene
Manson House, 26 Portland Place, London W1N 4EY

St Dunstan's (for Men and Women Blinded on War Service)
PO Box 58, 191 Marylebone Road, London NW1 5QN

Samaritans
17 Uxbridge Road, Slough, Berks SL1 1SN

The Scottish Association for Mental Health
67 York Place, Edinburgh, EM1 3ND

Scottish Epilepsy Association
(Seaborn Industries) 48 Govan Road, Glasgow G51 1JL

Scottish National Federation for the Welfare of the Blind
8 St Leonard's Rock, Perth PH2 8EB

Sesame
Christchurch, 27 Blackfriars Road, London SE1 8NY

The Spastics Society
12 Park Crescent, London W1N 4EQ

Terrence Higgins Trust
BM Aids, London WC1N 3XX

Toy Libraries Association
Seabrooke House, Wyllots Manor, Darkes Lane, Potters Bar,
Herts EN6 5MC

Index

Page references in *italics* refer to figures whereas those in **bold type** refer to tables.